# MANAGING ORAL HEALTHCARE DELIVERY:

## A RESOURCE FOR
## DENTAL PROFESSIONALS

# MANAGING ORAL HEALTHCARE DELIVERY:
## A RESOURCE FOR DENTAL PROFESSIONALS

Catherine L. Ganssle, R.D.H., M.S.

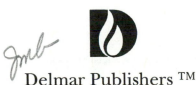

Delmar Publishers ™

I(T)P˙ An International Thomson Publishing Company

Albany • Bonn • Boston • Cincinnati • Detroit • London • Madrid • Melbourne
Mexico City • New York • Pacific Grove • Paris • San Francisco • Singapore • Tokyo
Toronto • Washington

## NOTICE TO THE READER

Cover: Terri Ryan, Synergy Design

**Delmar Staff**

| | |
|---|---|
| Acquisitions Editors: | William Burgower/Kimberly Davies |
| Assistant Editor: | Debra M. Flis |
| Project Editor: | Melissa A. Conan |
| Production Coordinator: | Mary Ellen Black |
| Editorial Assistant: | Donna Leto |
| Production Services: | Publishers' Design and Production Services, Inc. |

COPYRIGHT © 1995
By Delmar Publishers
A division of International Thomson Publishing Company
The ITP logo is a trademark under license
Printed in the United States of America

For more information, contact:

Delmar Publishers
3 Columbia Circle, Box 15015
Albany, NY 12212-5015

International Thomson Publishing Europe
Berkshire House 168-173
High Holborn
London WC1V7AA
England

Thomas Nelson Australia
102 Dodds Street
South Melbourne, 3205
Victoria, Australia

Nelson Canada
1120 Birchmount Road
Scarborough, Ontario
Canada, M1K 5G4

International Thomson Editores
Campos Eliseos 385, Piso 7
Col Polanco
11560 Mexico D F Mexico

International Thomson Publishing GmbH
Königswinterer Strasse 418
53227 Bonn
Germany

International Thomson Publishing Asia
221 Henderson Road
#05-10  Henderson Building
Singapore 0315

International Thomson Publishing—Japan
Kyowa Building, 3F
2-2-1 Hirakawacho
Chiyoda-ku, Tokyo 102
Japan

1  2  3  4  5  6  7  8  9  10  XXX  01  00  99  98  97  96  95  94

**Library of Congress Cataloging-in-Publication Data**

Ganssle, Catherine L.
   Managing oral healthcare delivery: a resource for dental professionals / Catherine L. Ganssle.
      p.   cm.
   Includes index.
   ISBN 0-8273-5532-7
   1. Dental hygiene—Practice.  2. Dental offices—Management.  I. Title.
RK60.5.G36  1995
617.6'01'68—dc20

94-16965
CIP

*This book is dedicated to my friends and colleagues*
*in the American Dental Hygienists' Association,*
*who have made all things possible.*

# CONTRIBUTORS

**Catherine C. Davis**, R.D.H., Ph.D., Clinical Research Coordinator at Poudre Valley Hospital, Fort Collins, Colorado, and Associate Clinical Professor of Dental Hygiene at the University of Colorado Dental School.

**Beverly Entwistle**, R.D.H., M.P.H., Public Health Adviser for the Portland Area Office of the Indian Health Service.

**Gail N. Cross-Poline**, R.D.H., M.S., Associate Professor and Chair, Department of Dental Hygiene, University of Colorado School of Dentistry.

**Catherine L. Ganssle**, R.D.H., M.S., owner of Softaid, Inc., clinical dental hygienist and study nurse, Rivers Center Dental Associates.

**Candy B. Ross**, R.D.H., B.S., Director of Professional Relations, Teledyne Water Pik.

# CONTENTS

# PREFACE

This book is for dental hygienists and is about the oral healthcare delivery system and their management roles in it. Although private clinical practice is, for now at least, the heart of healthcare delivery, dental hygienists are also working in a variety of other professional capacities. Hygienists are business owners or employed as managers in many areas, including education, private practice, public health, and the healthcare products industry.

A number of textbooks for dental hygienists only touch on the management of this industry. This book focuses on management exclusively. The many roles of dental hygienists are inter-related; management touches all of them. This book can serve as a general reference for all types of oral healthcare delivery and for all hygienists, even if they are not strictly filling a business ownership or management function. People who know how to manage their own work have a means to controlling their careers.

General principles of business management are applicable in all fields, from industry to information technology to service. Dental hygiene and dental practice are the principal parts of the oral healthcare delivery system, a service industry. Most often, dental hygiene and dental practice are part of small business. This book begins with general principles of business management, including examples from nonhealthcare industries, and businesses large and small. In Part 2, the dental hygiene profit center in clinical practice, as well as the specifics of dental practice management, are examined. The final section examines the management functions of dental hygienists in roles other than clinical practice.

For many, this approach may be a new way of looking at oral healthcare delivery and the roles of dental hygienists. Hopefully, the reader will gain a new view of and broader perspective on the profession of dental hygiene. Ultimately, this can lead to greater career satisfaction among practitioners and improved oral healthcare delivery for clients.

## ACKNOWLEDGMENTS

I offer my deepest thanks to those who have made this book possible; to my husband and business partner, Jack Ganssle, who has persevered in the face of challenges that would have defeated me; to Joannie Elder, a talented engineer, business manager, and mother, for her advice in all her areas of expertise; to Bob, for sharing his legal advice and business acumen; to Manny Quinones, who reviewed Chapter 3, and to Isaac Carpenter, who has helped me through many a financial report. A special word of thanks also goes to all my employers and employees who, over the years, have shown me the best and the worst of business management.

## AUTHOR'S NOTE

It is often a sad fact of modern life that things are changing too fast to keep up with them. To help the reader keep up, I offer an explanation of the gender references in this text. In an effort to be equitable, and in defiance of the otherwise infallible *Chicago Manual of Style*, the gender of the third-person pronoun changes in each chapter. The odd numbered chapters use the feminine and the even numbered chapters use the masculine. This may also offer the reader some additional challenges in identifying gender stereotypes.

In a further effort to achieve linguistic equity, I have attempted to standardize the language used to refer to those served by the healthcare delivery system. They have been called, among other things, patients, customers, consumers, and clients. In this text, patients, customers, and consumers are referred to as clients. This is consistent with the framework for theory development of the American Dental Hygienists' Association and is commonly used in other healthcare fields, such as nursing. Client may refer to a company, group, or individual. It is also a term often associated with a more modern approach to healthcare, in which the client is a participant, not a passive patient just following orders.

# PART 1

# PRINCIPLES OF BUSINESS MANAGEMENT

---

*Oral healthcare delivery is a business. A well-run practice, one operating with economic efficiency, employee involvement, and a commitment to quality, delivers quality healthcare at affordable prices. Its service is of value to the clients and can improve their quality of life.*

*Achieving quality and efficiency requires that a practice be run as a business. Practitioners are often uncomfortable with this fact, preferring to believe that the practice exists only to serve the public. A healthcare practice should certainly minister to the public welfare, but if it does so at the expense of going out of business, where will its clients go for care? Quality and caring do not happen by accident. Careful management is required and is as much a part of oral healthcare delivery as good clinical services. Without it, good clinical services go to waste.*

*Part 1 covers general principles of business management. Most of the discussion could apply to any sort of business, from manufacturing to information technology. A manager's job is to see that the work gets done. This means planning, coordinating, and directing people, money, and resources, shared functions in most business settings. The specifics will vary, but almost every manager is concerned with planning, human resources (people), finance (money), and marketing to some extent.*

*Part 1 discusses management in many types of businesses, not just oral healthcare. Parts 2 and 3 of this text are specific to dental hygiene and dental practice, but the first step is to become familiar with general principles of business management.*

# CHAPTER 1

# Planning

---

## Objectives

After reading this chapter and completing the review questions, the reader should be able to:

- List three reasons why businesses need to plan.
- Describe the planning cycle.
- Describe each of the elements of a strategic plan.
- State the significance of evaluation.

---

This chapter is about planning—the why and how of planning. As Harold Laski once said, "We must plan our civilization or perish." Plan or perish certainly applies to business as much as to civilizations, for a business without a plan is going nowhere, except probably out of business. It is difficult or impossible to meet long-term goals without planning, and worse yet, the company may meet its goals and never even know it.

## THE PLANNING CYCLE

Planning is a continuous, cyclical process. Although you may set aside specific time each year or each quarter to formally plan, collecting data and evaluating performance continues year-round.

Planning models are almost as numerous as are businesses. The important point to remember about planning is that you need to do it. The details of how you plan will vary from business to business. More examples of the planning process in specific industries are found in Chapters 11 (education), 12 (oral healthcare product manufacturing), and 13 (public health). As a manager, you will choose the planning model that best fits your situation. Just as the plan needs revision, you may find that the planning process will need occasional revision. The process you use, however, is less important than coming up with a viable plan.

The basic planning model given here is an amalgam of many others. The elements of the strategic plan are as follows:

mission

goals

objectives

action plans

evaluation

These elements constitute a cycle, as illustrated in Figure 1.1, not a stepwise process with a beginning and an end. If your business is not using this process or you are new to it, begin with the big picture, the mission statement.

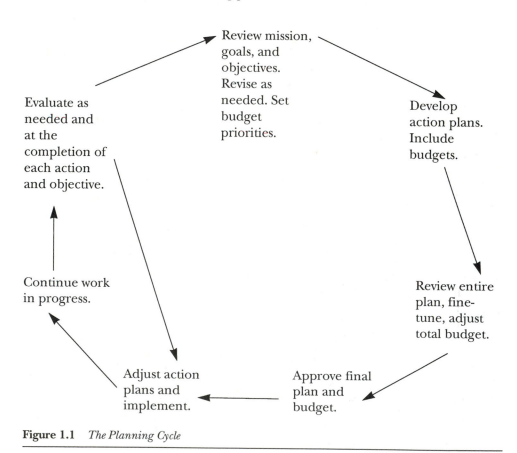

**Figure 1.1**   *The Planning Cycle*

The mission statement is ongoing and rarely changes. Goals are reviewed yearly, but they generally take longer than one or two years to achieve. Objectives for each goal are set yearly, although some objectives may take less than a year to achieve. Each objective encompasses a number of action plans, which are short term and explain how objectives will be realized and evaluated. Evaluations take place as specified in the action plans, and the overall strategic plan is reviewed yearly. Some businesses may need to evaluate and review quarterly.

How should the cycle coincide with the fiscal year? Although the calendar year begins in January and ends in December, many businesses begin and end their corporate (fiscal) years on a different twelve-month cycle—the federal government, for example, begins its year in October and ends in September. A discussion of fiscal year planning is beyond the scope of this text, but advanced courses in finance cover it. If you think you need to make a change, consult with a certified public accountant (CPA).

You will probably want to implement the strategic plan at the beginning of the fiscal year. In that case, you must adjust the planning cycle so that the action plans and associated budget are in final form and ready to go at the start of the fiscal year. This means that you will need to begin the preliminary work in sufficient time to complete all the steps by the end of the fiscal year. How long this will take will depend on the size of your organization and its existing procedures.

## Who Is Involved in Planning?

There are many points of view on this issue. Traditionally, planning was restricted to upper management. In a large corporation this might mean just the chief executive officer (CEO), president, and senior vice presidents. In a small business, such as a dental office, this might mean the dentists who own the practice and perhaps their associates. In many, many cases, this type of management approach has failed.

In the past two decades, it has become customary to involve many levels in management decisions. Management by objectives (MBO) may have seen its heyday, but it is a model with elements well worth considering. Managing by objectives generally means involving middle managers and employees in setting objectives and determining evaluation mechanisms. One of its major advantages is that those involved in creating objectives are more likely to feel that they "own" the objectives and will work hard to achieve them. In the following discussion, you will see many points at which employees can become involved in the planning process.

Walter Wriston (1990), a former chairman of Citicorp and "one of America's most respected managers," offered some sound advice about what the job of a manager is: "The job of the manager today: find the best people you can, motivate them, and allow them to do the job their own way."

You and your management team will have to decide who, within your company or practice, to include in the planning process. You may need to make adjustments along the way. In general, though, the more people you include, the more creative, innovative ideas you will get and the more those people will be motivated to work within the plan.

## Budgeting and Planning

Budgeting is best considered as part of the planning cycle. Developing the budget as you develop the plan will result in a plan you can afford to implement. In a small business, it should be possible to do this. By contrast, in a large, complex organization, the budgeting process may be somewhat separate from the strategic planning process and allowances for revisions of the plan and the budget, as both evolve, will be necessary.

## Situation Analysis

Don't forget to consider the total situation when planning. Conduct a situation analysis, considering your organization's internal strengths and weaknesses, as well as threats and opportunities from sources outside the company. Build upon the organization's strong points and work to improve them. Just like your teeth, if you ignore them, they may go away. Plan to strengthen or eliminate your weaknesses. Don't ignore them. Consider what is happening in the business environment: the economic trends, the changes in the community, your competitors and their products. Look for opportunities to enter new markets or to offer new products or services. What is happening that could threaten the plan, damage the company, or erode your market? Things are everchanging, and you need to accommodate this fact in your planning.

Cohen (1990) had this to say about risk:

> Never be afraid to take risks. If you work for someone else, taking risks is part of what you are getting paid for. If you work for yourself, it is the only way you can become successful.

As a manager, taking risks is something you must do, but you don't have to be irresponsible about it. Make it part of your plan.

# MISSION

Every business needs a mission. A mission statement is broad, takes a long-range view, and discusses what the business does and why it exists. Unfortunately, not every business has a mission statement, although most corporations must include something similar in their original incorporation papers. Every business, including a dental or dental hygiene practice, needs a mission statement. Management and employees need to know "why"—why the business exists, where it's going, what its purpose is. Without this focal point, it is difficult to proceed. How can you get there if you don't know where you're going?

If your business has a mission statement, review it periodically as part of the strategic planning process. Occasionally—*not* yearly—the mission statement may need revision. It should be revised only when the purpose of the business changes, and this won't happen often, if at all.

What's in a mission statement? Some corporate mission statements are several paragraphs long and others are only one sentence. The mission statement should be long enough to state the purpose of the organization clearly, but concise enough to keep the meaning clear.

## Examples

The following is the mission statement of the American Dental Hygienists' Association, a nonprofit corporation. Can you tell from this statement what the purpose of the ADHA is? If you were part of the management team, would this statement give you a point of reference for moving the organization forward in the right direction?

> To improve the public's total health, the mission of the American Dental Hygienists' Association is to advance the art and science of dental hygiene by increasing the awareness of and ensuring access to quality oral healthcare, promoting the highest standards of dental hygiene education, licensure and practice, and representing and promoting the interests of dental hygienists.

The ADHA clearly intends that its efforts on behalf of the profession of dental hygiene will benefit the public as well as dental hygienists. The organization's focus, however, is on service to its members, as is usual with this type of business.

The following is the mission statement of a small, high-technology electronics firm. You should be able to read it and know why this business exists. As with many high-tech firms, the product line will change over time, often dramatically, often rapidly. Will this mission statement provide the necessary direction in such a volatile market?

> We will be a responsive, reliable company that is a pleasure to do business with. This includes quality products, superb literature/documentation, efficient lead fulfillment, accurate and friendly pre-sale fielding of technical/sales questions, quick and easy access to sales and demo units, and unparalleled post-sale support.

Although this statement strongly declares how the company will do business, it does not state clearly why the business exists. The owners most likely assume that the business exists to make a profit, but it might be wise to make this purpose clear when sharing the mission statement with employees. This mission statement, although out of the ordinary, does provide management and employees with the direction they need to continue with strategic planning. Regardless of changes in the marketplace or product line, this mission statement will provide long-term focus for all company activities.

The following is the mission statement of a dental practice. Does this mission statement tell the managers, employees, clients, and you what type of practice this is? If you were the practice manager, would this statement give you the information you need to proceed with the strategic plan, to develop goals, objectives, and action plans?

> Our purpose is to serve our patients. We will provide them with the best possible care, in a safe, friendly, cooperative environment.

This mission statement puts service and quality right up front. Safety, friendliness, and cooperation can apply to patients as well as employees. Although this mission statement could be a little longer and more specific, it clearly states the priorities of the practice.

# GOALS

Goals should be firm. They are statements of what an organization wants to achieve. Goals should also be broad—not specific—and obtainable. This does not mean that they should be obtained easily or quickly, for they may take years to achieve. The purpose of planning is to make goals achievable. If goals are not attainable, the plan will seem useless.

Avoid goals that require more than about 10 years to achieve. In most business environments today, change happens so rapidly that the extremely long-range goal you set today may be meaningless 10 or 20 years from now, even if you do reach it. Focusing goals on the near future will facilitate creating realistic objectives. A business may indeed have things to accomplish in 20 or 50 or 100 years, but such long-range goals will be difficult to plan for specifically now. The solution to a very long range "wish" is to break it down into several pieces and work toward a goal attainable in 5 or 10 years.

## Examples

The following are examples of goals. Note that although they state clearly what is to be accomplished, they are not specific about how or when.

A personal goal might be to "obtain a bachelor's degree." Many factors might be involved in reaching this goal, including finances, grades, and housing.

An example of a corporate goal is to "take the company public." In other words, a privately owned corporation intends to become publicly owned by offering stock for sale on a public stock market, such as the New York Stock Exchange. Many, very specific objectives and requirements are involved in achieving such a goal.

A goal for a dental practice might be to "provide preventive oral healthcare for the citizens of Smallville." The supporting objectives will need to be more specific. Probably not all of the citizens of Smallville will seek treatment in this one practice. It may take considerable time to develop the preventive program and to market it successfully.

Goals tell management what to do. Objectives define in quantitative terms, with deadlines, what steps are necessary to reach the goals.

# OBJECTIVES

Objectives are flexible. Achieving one goal requires reaching a number of objectives, and reaching all the objectives could take several years. Objectives can be steps to a goal, requiring completion of step 1 before continuing to step 2, and so on. Or work can proceed on objectives concurrently.

Objectives are specific. They should include three components: an action word, a result or level of performance, and a time frame for completion. Your goals may be somewhat nebulous and, in the long run, you may not reach them. Remember that objectives should be obtainable. Never write objectives that are far beyond the abilities of the business resources to achieve.

For example, a well-written objective is "to control 50% of the soft drink market in the United States by the third quarter of 1998." But such an objective might not be obtainable. If you are a small business with 30 employees and a $2 million dollar budget and you're competing against Coca-Cola, you definitely need a more realistic objective.

## Examples

In reaching the personal goal "to obtain a bachelor's degree," one objective might be "to get a $2000 scholarship from the United Negro College Fund before the fall semester." There is an action (to get), a specific result ($2000 scholarship), and a deadline (fall semester).

To "take the company public," one objective might be "to prepare an audited yearly financial statement." There is an action (to prepare), a specific result (an audited financial statement), and an implied deadline (yearly). You would need to accomplish this objective for several years prior to taking the company public. You should include it in the strategic plan because considerable time and expense are involved in preparing audited financial statements. In a large corporation, this procedure is probably ongoing, part of normal operations, and as such might not be a specific objective. Many other objectives must be ongoing concurrently with this one. Going public requires more than just having audited financial statements. It means that work must begin on the other objectives at the same time so that everything will be ready in time.

For the dental practice that wants to "provide preventive oral healthcare for the citizens of Smallville," an objective might be "to increase senior citizen participation in our preventive program by 25% by December 1998." There is an action (to increase participation), a specific result (by 25%), and a time frame (by December 1998). The practice must accomplish an objective to develop the "preventive program" before working on this objective.

Objectives tell management what must be accomplished and when. Action plans describe how this will be done and what resources (time, people, or money) are involved.

## ACTION PLANS

Just as one goal may need a number of objectives, one objective may involve several action plans. Action plans specify details. They state what steps are involved in the action, who is responsible for each step, what resources are required, and how much time is required for each step. Action plans can change. Although developing action plans is part of the strategic planning process, it will probably be necessary to change some action plans or develop new ones during the planning cycle, not just at one time of the year. When writing action plans, be sure to allow for this flexibility in the plan. Have alternatives on hand.

Begin by brainstorming. Get together whatever group you have decided to work with and spend some time writing down all the ideas that come to mind. List all the actions that might help achieve the objective. Don't edit the comments or discuss their merits during the brainstorming session(s). You may want to involve more than one group or different individuals at this stage. Just get all the ideas out.

This is also a good time to discuss strengths and weaknesses, opportunities and threats, but don't get bogged down in the analysis. Remember, you need an *action* plan. If you let the group spend all its time on analysis, you won't get around to action. Take both the internal and external environments into account in your planning, but don't let this control your thinking.

The next step, probably working with a smaller group, is to discuss the alternatives and choose the action or actions best suited to reaching the objectives within the limits of your available resources. Don't choose too many actions, or you'll spend all your time planning. Save the ideas you don't work on for use for alternative plans or during the next planning cycle.

After you have settled on a limited number of actions that clearly support the objective, develop a plan for *each* action. Work on one action plan at a time per group, and be very specific in developing the plan. State clearly who will be responsible for which activities and who will work on them, and state when activities are to be completed. The reason for committing to a deadline is to ensure that the task is accomplished on time. Include a list of materials, equipment, space, or other resources needed to complete the action if any of these are needed.

Be specific about budget requirements. Getting the budget right may involve a lot of give and take. Part of the planning process is deciding how much of the available money goes to which objectives and which action plans. If there are a number of groups doing the planning, they must coordinate their use of resources. Budget limitations are common. Some of your alternative plans may include provisions for limited funds or loss of personnel.

## Examples

Action plans for the objective of producing audited financial statements might include actions for contracting with an accounting firm, evaluating existing accounting methods, installing a new computer-based accounting system, and streamlining in-house financial reporting procedures. Each of these actions would be detailed in a separate action plan.

Refer to Figure 1.2, an action plan for the objective of producing audited financial statements. The action is to review the current bookkeeping system and software. The deadline for completion of the action is listed just below the action, with the total budget for the action plan listed just below the deadline. You will notice that two people, Graham and Kristina, are working on this action plan concurrently. Each has start and end dates for the steps for which he or she is responsible. Most of the budget amounts are the accounting rates for Graham's and Kristina's time, which is what the company estimates it costs to keep each of them working per hour. The budget also includes rates for meeting with the accountants and with the computer consultant but not for the CFO and the bookkeepers. Their time will be included with general overhead.

Objective: Prepare an audited yearly financial statement.
Action: Evaluate the current bookkeeping system and software.
Deadline: June 3 , 1995
Total budget: $1500

| Steps | Responsible | Start | End | Budget |
|---|---|---|---|---|
| 1. Document present bookkeeping methods. | Graham | 5/1/95 | 5/12/95 | $270 |
| a. Interview CFO. | Graham | 5/1/95 | 5/1/95 | .5 hr @ $30/hr |
| b. Interview bookkeeper. | Graham | 5/2/95 | 5/2/95 | .5 hr @ $30/hr |
| c. Review accting manual. | Graham | 5/3/95 | 5/8/95 | 4 hr @ $30/hr |
| d. Write summary. | Graham | 5/9/95 | 5/11/95 | 4 hr @ $30/hr |
| 2. Document capabilities of present financial software. | Kristina | 5/1/95 | 5/12/95 | $305 |
| a. Interview CFO. | Kristina | 5/2/95 | 5/2/95 | .5 hr @ $35/hr |
| b. Interview bookkeeper. | Kristina | 5/3/95 | 5/3/95 | .5 hr @ $35/hr |
| c. Interview computer consultant. | Kristina | 5/4/95 | 5/4/95 | 1 hr @ $95/hr |
| d. Review software documentation. | Kristina | 5/5/95 | 5/9/95 | 4 hr @ $35/hr |
| e. Write summary. | Kristina | 5/10/95 | 5/11/95 | 4 hr @ $35/hr |
| 3. Review present methods and capabilities with accountants. | Graham, Kristina | 5/15/95 | 5/15/95 | $555 |
| a. Meet with accountants to present summaries for their review. | Graham, Kristina | 5/15/95 | 5/15/95 | 2 hr @ $165/hr |
| b. Gather addtl info; answer accountants' questions. | Graham | 5/25/95 | 5/30/95 | 2 hr @ $30/hr |
| c. Meet w/accountants to discuss necessary changes. | Graham, Kristina | 5/31/95 | 5/31/95 | 1 hr @ $165/hr |
| 4. Work with CFO to develop action plan for modifying existing systems. | Kristina | 6/1/95 | 6/2/95 | $200 |

**Figure 1.2** *Example action plan*

Refer to Figure 1.3. It is an action plan for the objective of getting a $2000 scholarship from the United Negro College Fund before the fall semester. The action, to complete the application, differs in format from the first example: It is less formal, since it is only intended for personal use. The student is responsible for all the action steps, and the budget is 0 because no one is paying for the student's time while she does the work. There is a column for resources because she needs to plan to make these resources available.

Objective:      Get a $2000 scholarship from the United Negro College Fund before the fall semester.
Action:         Complete the application
Deadline:     Feb. 1, 1995
Total budget:   $5 (postage and copies as needed)

| Steps | Responsible | Start | End | Resources |
|---|---|---|---|---|
| 1. Meet with financial aid office. | Self | 10/2/95 | 10/2/95 | Ms. Rogers |
| 2. Gather and forward transcripts. | " | 10/2/95 | 11/3/95 | |
| 3. Gather parents' financial data. | " | 10/14/95 | 10/15/95 | Parents |
| 4. Gather recommendations. | " | 10/2/95 | 11/3/95 | Dr. Hanover<br>L. Bauer<br>T. Singer |
| 5. Complete first draft of application. | " | 11/4/95 | 11/4/95 | |
| 6. Type final draft of application. | | 11/13/95 | 11/13/95 | Typewriter |
| 7. Mail application. | | 11/14/95 | 11/14/95 | |

**Figure 1.3**   *Example action plan*

Figure 1.4 is a blank action planning form. It combines features of both Figures 1.2 and 1.3. Several different examples of action plan formats have been presented, but each organization must develop an action plan format that best suits its needs or the requirements of specific projects or departments.

## EVALUATION

Evaluation is not a final step. It must be an ongoing process. Each action plan should contain evaluation components—who, when, where, how much, and by when. The actions should certainly be evaluated when completed, but the person primarily responsible should stay in touch with the process to be sure that the plan is on track and can be completed as specified and on time. Of course, this doesn't always happen. Plans may need adjustment or replacement. Be prepared.

Evaluate the overall strategic plan regularly, at the same time each year. The objectives contain evaluation components. At the time of the yearly evaluation, discuss whether you have achieved each objective, why or why not, what worked and what didn't. Objectives may require modification based on the evaluation, the situation analysis, or because they have been completed.

The importance of evaluation cannot be overemphasized. Without it, you may have no idea whether your plan is working beautifully or falling apart around you. Evaluations should be as objective as possible. Avoid the temptation to finger-point. Although it is helpful to know what went wrong and why, nothing will be accomplished by focusing only on the past, or by publicly berating those responsible for errors. Find out what went wrong, and plan to correct the problem as quickly as possible.

| Steps | Responsible | Resources | Start | End | Budget |
|-------|-------------|-----------|-------|-----|--------|
|       |             |           |       |     |        |
|       |             |           |       |     |        |
|       |             |           |       |     |        |
|       |             |           |       |     |        |
|       |             |           |       |     |        |
|       |             |           |       |     |        |
|       |             |           |       |     |        |
|       |             |           |       |     |        |
|       |             |           |       |     |        |
|       |             |           |       |     |        |
|       |             |           |       |     |        |
|       |             |           |       |     |        |
|       |             |           |       |     |        |

**Figure 1.4**  *Example action planning form*

focus ➤━━━━━━━━➤ communicate ➤━━━━━━━━➤ achieve

**Figure 1.5**

## *Summary*

The planning cycle involves the development or revision of a strategic plan, including a mission statement, goals, objectives, action plans, and a budget, implementation of the plan, and ongoing evaluation. Businesses must plan to succeed, even if some get by for a while with no planning. A plan will give an organization focus. A business that is focused can communicate what to do and how and get everyone focused on working for the plan—and in this way can achieve results (see Figure 1.5).

## *Review Questions*

1. Write a mission statement for an organization in which you are involved. This could be your dental hygiene association, college or university, or community group.

2. Find out whether the organization you wrote about in Question 1 has an existing mission statement. If so, how does yours compare?

3. Write a personal goal, with objectives and action plans for yourself. Choose a goal you really want to achieve.

4. Write an objective to go with the goal of the dental practice to "provide preventive oral healthcare for the citizens of Smallville."

5. Briefly describe the Smallville Dental Group. Include a description of the community of Smallville, what type of practice the dental group is, and how many employees it has. Now write a doable action plan to support the objective you wrote in Question 4. If you really want a challenge, include budget information.

**SUGGESTED READING**

DeBono, E. (1970). *Lateral thinking: Creativity step by step.* New York: Harper & Row.

Naisbitt, J., & Aburdene, P. (1990). *Megatrends 2000.* New York: William Morrow & Co.

Tzu, S. (1989). *The art of war.* Translated by T. Cleary. Boston: Shambhala Publications.

**REFERENCES**

Wriston, W. (1990). The state of American management. *Harvard Business Review*, 68(1), 78–83.

Cohen, W. A. (1990). *The art of the leader.* New Jersey: Prentice-Hall, p. iv.

# CHAPTER 2

# Human Resources

## Objectives

After reading this chapter and completing the review questions, the reader should be able to:

- List at least three reasons why it is important to have written policies and procedures and to follow them.
- Recognize key risk management issues.
- Define the manager's role in recruitment, hiring, and termination.
- Recognize costs associated with staff turnover.
- List the three components to include in performance evaluation objectives.

## LEADERSHIP

You can be a successful leader without being a successful manager, but you will never be a successful manager without being a good leader. Many excellent references on leadership are available. Kotter (1990), in "What Leaders Really Do," sums up the differences between management and leadership: "Leadership complements management; it doesn't replace it." Leaders direct change by developing a vision—managers plan and budget to cope with complexity. Leaders align people—managers organize and staff. Leaders motivate and inspire—managers problem solve. In your role as a human resource manager, you will certainly be involved with planning, budgeting, organizing, staffing, and problem solving. If, at the same time, you can create a vision, align people, and inspire them to make the vision a reality, your job will be much easier. You will be a leader among managers.

It is important to recognize that management skills and leadership skills differ in important ways and so need to be developed differently. Management is a job, one that usually follows established company structure, whereas leadership may be unofficial. As such, leaders may not fit the hierarchical structure of a company, yet most companies will prosper if they have positive, motivated leadership within. Part of your management responsibilities is to foster both management and leadership development in your employees. Their management training may be official and regular, while their leadership development, and yours, will require behind-the-scenes work, possibly in areas outside the work setting.

Hard-and-fast rules may apply in human resource management, but they change frequently. What you say and do can be highly structured. When managing complexity, leadership is necessary to direct change.

## POLICIES AND PROCEDURES

Every organization, no matter how small, has some employment procedures. They may not be consistent and they may not be written, but there is some usual way of doing things. The larger and more complex the organization becomes, the more codified the procedures become. Such structure can be beneficial if it enhances job performance and consistency. It can be detrimental if people do things just because they're SOP (standard operating procedure), without considering to what makes sense and what works best. It is especially important that all employment procedures be applied consistently.

The terms *policy* and *procedure* are often used interchangeably, but they do have different connotations. According to Webster's dictionary, policy is "a principle chosen to guide decision making." Procedure, according to Webster's, is "a certain way of getting things done." In companies that make a distinction, policies are broad and often require executive approval for modification, and procedures would be the "how to" guidelines for routine tasks, such as how to get approval for vacation leave or how to fill out your time card. To simplify this discussion, these terms are used interchangeably. Be sure that within your work setting, however, you use the terms to be consistent with the rest of the company.

The manager's role in policies and procedures is twofold. Managers are involved at some level in creating or modifying policies and procedures and are responsible for seeing that established policies and procedures are followed.

As we discussed in Chapter 1, it is generally best to involve as many levels of employees as possible in management decisions. This is true in the establishment of company policies and procedures, for which most employees will have some very definite opinions, for example, on sick leave and vacation pay. Although all won't have it their way, all should be given input, for those doing the job have the best understanding of how to get it done. Employees may not have the big picture of how their work relates to other procedures, however, and this is what management provides.

## RISK MANAGEMENT

Risk management refers to minimizing legal risks. Although it is not possible to prevent all types of legal entanglements, you can take steps to reduce the company's legal exposure. This is risk management.

In large organizations, company policies should be written, especially those relating to employment practices, in order to apply them consistently. In small businesses, employing about 20 or fewer people, it may not be necessary to have written policies. In fact, there may be some advantage to not having written policies. It would leave management much more flexibility in dealing with unusual situations. Even in the absence of written policies, it is important that your actions be consistent. Failure to have legally sound, established employment procedures and to practice them with absolute consistency can lead to significant legal problems. If your business has a policy manual or employee handbook, it should be reviewed regularly, with legal advice, and be kept up to date and concurrent with laws at the federal, state, and even local level that affect business operation. This chapter is a general discussion of employment procedures. It is no substitute for legal advice specific to your state and business.

If your business needs to develop a written policy or procedure manual, prewritten policy manuals, some specific to your business or industry, are available and can be adapted to your business fairly easily. Once again, laws vary considerably from place to place. Even if you begin with a published template, the finished manual needs to be reviewed by an attorney familiar with the employment laws affecting your business and location.

Some statements in a policy manual may be interpreted as a contract between the employer and the employee. To avoid misinterpretation, initially state that the manual is not a contract and that employees are employees-at-will unless they have a specific contract with the employer. These guidelines are not directly applicable to managing unionized employees (organized labor). There is little flexibility in defining policies and procedures specific to union members, as they are negotiated with the union and can be changed only through official channels.

## CONTENT OF A POLICY OR PROCEDURE MANUAL

Here is a sample outline for a policy manual. A policy or procedure manual should be regarded as a dynamic document—that is, one that is expected to change often. Produce the manual with an in-office word processor, rather than having it typed manually with each revision sent for outside printing, so it is accessible and can be updated easily.

Some of the sections listed may not apply to small business. There may be additional items needed for specific industries. Chapter 7 includes specific information relative to managing oral healthcare delivery.

### Rules and Regulations

This section can contain general guidelines for the work environment and may include such things as a nonsmoking policy. It may also include a list of serious offenses, such as theft of company property or possession of a weapon on company property, for which there are serious consequences, such as immediate dismissal. A code of ethics might be included in this section or listed separately.

## Occupational Safety and Health

Depending on the work environment, this may be a required section in the policy manual. Some settings, however, such as a dental office, where the rules are extensive, might need a separate manual to comply with specific standards. There are safety and health guidelines for most work settings, usually set by state standards, but also influenced by federal and local regulations.

## Worker's Compensation

Worker's compensation is a government-sponsored benefit for which most employees are eligible. Including information about worker's comp in the policy manual is beneficial, and employers are also usually required to post notices (which are sent by the government agency responsible) in conspicuous areas in the work place. Employees who suffer a job-related injury may be eligible for benefits under the worker's comp plan. Regulations vary from state to state.

As is the case with unemployment insurance, worker's compensation is financed in part by employer contributions, based on payroll. Worker's comp can be a significant expense for businesses. California, for example, allows generous worker's compensation payments and qualifies for payment not just physical injuries but also job-related stress. Employers' contributions have risen to such an extent that many small businesses have been forced to close and large employers, most notably automobile manufacturers, have moved their operations to other states. Regardless of location, it is best, not just from an ethical standpoint, but from a practical one, to keep employees safe and free from injury.

Many industries use employee-led safety teams to reduce accidents and injury. As with other aspects of management, such employee involvement motivates them to take responsibility for all aspects of their work and work environment, improve quality, reduce problems, and free managers for other responsibilities.

## Attendance and Punctuality

Although regular arrival and departure times might vary from employee to employee, this section would give the details of companywide policy on such topics as the correct procedure to call in sick and the specific consequences for habitual tardiness. Because some people leave their jobs without ever officially giving notice, this section should include a statement to the effect that after a certain number of consecutive workdays missed, the employee will be considered to have voluntarily quit.

## Payroll

Specify what the paydays are, for example, every other Friday or the first and fifteenth of the month. Explain payroll deductions for social security taxes, unemployment insurance, worker's compensation insurance, and federal and state income taxes. The company pays more than the employee contribution for social security taxes, unemployment insurance, and worker's compensation insurance. Often, employees don't realize this fact and fail to understand just how much the business spends to keep them employed. This section can explain employer tax contributions and might also state the procedures to follow for payroll or tax questions, necessary changes, or disputes.

There may be payroll deductions for health insurance, life or disability insurance, or contributions to retirement plans. These benefits should be explained in detail in other areas of the policy manual, but it is a good idea to mention any applicable deductions in the payroll section so that employees can interpret their payroll checks by referring to this one place.

## Hours of Work

This section might list regular office hours. If the company has a flextime policy, this is a good place to explain it. Flextime programs allow employees to begin and end their workdays at times of their own choosing. For example, regular office hours may be eight to five, but some employees may choose to work seven to four. Although it is highly unlikely that any private dental practice would use flextime, this practice is common in many federal government offices. Usually employees have to choose their flexhours and stick to them, not change from day to day. Clearly state the procedure and mechanisms for change.

## Overtime or Compensation Time

Most businesses follow the guidelines established by the Fair Labor Standards Act (FLSA) in classifying all job positions as either exempt or nonexempt. Nonexempt employees are paid hourly and may be eligible for overtime pay. Salaried, or exempt, employees usually do not receive overtime pay, but they may be eligible for compensation time, if you have such a program. Exempt employees are exempt from some provisions of the FLSA, while nonexempt employees are not. Check with your personnel office or legal counsel to see how the FLSA applies to your business and industry. If you are responsible for managing union personnel, be sure that you understand their employment guidelines and follow them. Union policies and procedures will probably be contained in a separate section or manual.

Overtime policy should state who is eligible to receive overtime pay, what the pay rate is (usually time and half or double time), what the procedure is for authorizing overtime, and what constitutes overtime (working, for example, more than 40 hours in a workweek).

In some companies, exempt employees, who are not eligible for overtime pay, may accrue compensation time for working more than the standard workweek (35 or 40 hours, whatever the company policy is). Compensation time, or personal leave time, is usually accrued at the rate of 1/2 hour for every hour of overtime worked. The policy manual should also state what the maximum accrual is, for example, 24 hours per fiscal quarter, and how it may be taken (all at once or no more than one day at a time maximum).

## Holiday Schedule

This section should contain a list of company holidays for which employees will be paid. The policy might also delineate who is eligible for holiday pay. Typically, employees on unpaid leave do not receive holiday pay, but employees on paid leave do. Part-time employees may not be eligible for holiday pay at all, or only if a holiday falls on one of their regularly scheduled workdays. This is often an issue in private dental practice. Delineating a policy and applying it consistently can prevent misunderstandings.

## Leave

There are many types of leave: annual (vacation), personal, sick, military, leaves of absence (medical or personal), and jury duty. Personal leave and sick leave are sometimes combined into one category. The policy manual should define each category, how it is accrued, how it can be used, and how and when to get approval for taking it. Annual leave and personal leave often allow some maximum accrual amount before being lost. For example, the company might have a policy that any vacation leave remaining at the end of a two-year period will be lost. If an employee could accrue three weeks of vacation leave per year, at the end of the second year the employee would have six weeks of vacation. For a key employee to be gone even this long might be hard for the rest of the staff.

## Benefits

The company might choose to offer plans from among a myriad of benefits: health, disability, or life insurance; profit-sharing, pension, or retirement plans; educational assistance; free parking; or uniform allowance. There are many others, depending on employee interest and company resources. The policy manual should explain each program in detail, stating who is eligible, how benefits are administered, and the procedures to follow when questions or problems arise. Benefits may also be negotiated individually with employees, and all employees may not receive all available benefits. Each benefit option might require a section of its own in the policy manual.

   Laws and regulations covering employee benefits also vary depending on business structure. For example, an incorporated business is often required to offer all benefits on an equal basis to all employees, although corporate officers may be an exception. Unincorporated businesses, such as partnerships or sole proprietorships, may be exempt from some of these requirements. Additionally, it is common practice for companies to arrange employee benefits packages such that the benefits are untaxable. The laws regarding benefits plans and taxes are complex and changing. Consult with a certified public accountant (CPA) or other knowledgeable professional when designing a benefits package.

## Technology

Most modern offices contain at least one computer and so should have policies on managing technology. One of the most common areas of concern is the prevention of computer system contamination by computer viruses. The procedures for importing data or software into the company computer or computer system should be specific (developed with the advice of an expert) and followed carefully. For many industries, in-house information is vital and must not be lost or destroyed, by viruses or negligence. If your business stores many important records on the computer(s), you will probably also need procedures for regularly backing up the data. The policy manual should describe other technology procedures that must be applied companywide.

# STAFFING

Even very small, technology-oriented businesses, where machines or computers perform most of the operations, must employ some living human beings to interface with the outside world. If all a company's employees disappeared or were incompetent, no amount of technology could keep the company afloat. The staff is the heart of any business. Customers may be the lifeblood of a business, but no manager can afford to take employees for granted. Staffing is a dynamic process. Even in a stable firm with little turnover, you need to keep an eye on all areas of staffing, including recruitment, termination, and evaluation. If you are a manager in a small business, you will probably be responsible for personnel yourself. In a large organization, there may be a personnel or human resources department to handle some of these items. In the end, though, you will be responsible for how work gets done in your area of responsibility and so you should be aware of staffing procedures, even if they are not directly your responsibility.

## Recruitment

The time to begin recruitment efforts is not when an employee leaves. If you do that, you're already behind. Who will train the new hire? Who will do the work of the recently departed employee while you search for a replacement? Of course, you can't have a replacement waiting in the wings for every employee, but you can have ongoing recruitment and staff development activities that will make it faster and cheaper to fill vacancies. If there are management levels reporting to you, those managers need to be active recruiters as well.

There can be various reasons for taking on new employees. One is expansion; an area may be growing and need new personnel to handle the additional work load. Planning for staff increases (or reductions) should be part of your strategic planning process. As you coordinate the action plans within the overall strategic plan, management should be able to predict where staff changes will be needed and cope with unexpected events. A stable work force will strengthen employee morale and public relations, whereas high staff turnover may leave clients or the business community with the impression that your company is unstable.

While it is great to be expanding and hiring new employees, be careful not to expand your staff too rapidly to accommodate the change. Your staffing projections need to be long range, beyond one quarter or one year. You do not want to hire ten new people in January, only to discover you have to fire five of them in

December when you finish a project. Additionally, the costs associated with staff turnover can be significant. (See Associated Costs, page 31.)

There are two sources of new staff members—external and internal. External hires would be those brought in from outside the company. If you are in a small business or one that is expanding rapidly, all your new staff may be from outside the company. There may simply not be enough personnel within the organization to recruit from one project or department to another. There may not even be departments. In a larger company, the staff may indeed be large enough that people can change jobs within the company.

When filling management positions, consider promoting from within. In other words, make every effort to fill upper-level jobs from within the company. Employees like to see that they have advancement opportunities within the company and need not change firms in order to advance. Promoting from within improves morale, facilitates recruitment, and reduces training costs. Unfortunately, such promotions are not always possible. Your company may not have an employee qualified to be promoted for a particular job, or it may have a very flat structure so that there is no movement up a corporate ladder because there is no corporate ladder. This may be by choice or because you have a very small organization.

## INTERNAL RECRUITMENT

Internal recruitment can be a tricky business. Offering employees mobility, both lateral and vertical, within your organization is fine, but never gut or demoralize one department or group to fill vacancies in another. This can be avoided through careful planning and internal communication during the planning process, by defining where staff cutbacks will be necessary and identifying other areas of the company where, with minimal re-training, those people can be relocated. Retraining a qualified current employee for a new position is usually more cost effective than training an outsider with no experience with your company or clients.

A good reason for staying in touch with employees within your company, even those for whom you are not directly responsible, is that you will be aware of their capabilities. The perfect person to fill a vacancy in your area may be in the office down the hall. Keeping in touch is an important part of recruitment. Internally, this means networking informally within your company, getting to know other employees at all levels, and letting them know about the work that your group does. Be positive when speaking about your area of responsibility. You never know when you may want to hire the person you are talking to, so focus on the best. "Never criticize, condemn or complain" (Carnegie, 1981).

## EXTERNAL RECRUITMENT

External recruitment can be costly. The costs may include advertising, travel (for you or prospective employees), legal advice, or, the one most often overlooked: the time spent screening, interviewing, and checking references. Hiring through an employment agency will save on advertising, travel, screening, interviewing, and checking references, but you can expect to pay the agency as much as 20% of the new hire's annual salary as a placement fee.

There are advantages to going through an employment agency, however. Depending on your business and location, if a lot of advertising and interviewing is required to fill a position, you may spend well over 20% of the new hire's annual salary on recruitment and placement. Another potential cost of recruitment, discussed further under Associated Costs (p. 31), is termination. Suppose you hire the wrong person because there wasn't time or money available to check references carefully or to bring in someone better qualified from out of town to interview? If you have to fire this employee during or shortly after training, your company will have invested quite a bit on the wrong person. Suppose you can't fire the "mistake" because there is no more money in the budget for recruitment? What will it cost you in lost customers or lost sales or lawsuits to keep the wrong person on the job?

An employment agency or professional recruiter can help you avoid these pitfalls. They are in the employment business and so distribute the advertising and other recruitment costs over many placements. They may have steady regional or national contacts and therefore have more access to qualified personnel than you do.

If you do use an agency, negotiate the placement fees and guarantee (the amount of time the new hire must remain with the company before the placement fee must be paid). In a down economy, with many people unemployed, you will have the advantage. In a market where workers are in high demand, you may have to pay more, but having a recruitment advantage may be worth the price.

There are good reasons to hire through agencies, but many companies will not use them. If managers are constantly keeping up with recruitment, it should be possible to successfully and cost effectively hire new staff members without agency help.

A great source of applicants for entry-level positions is schools. The nature of your business will determine the schools from which you recruit. In oral health-care delivery, local or regional dental hygiene or dental schools are a good source and will probably welcome your involvement in alumni associations or other school activities. High schools and trade schools may be sources of applicants for nonprofessional positions. In fact, many school systems encourage partnership programs with area businesses. Your business participation in these programs would make a significant contribution to the community, be good public relations, and can help in employment recruiting. If a partnership program doesn't exist, consider initiating one.

As mentioned in the internal recruitment section, successful managers stay in touch, even with external sources. There are many ways to do this, depending on the exact nature of your business. You need to be a part of the network for your profession or business and to maintain contacts within your community, within your professional organization, management organization, and local Chamber of Commerce or social groups

Never say anything about any employee of your company that you would not want made public. If you wouldn't feel comfortable seeing your remark on the front page of the paper, don't say it, or you may be exposing yourself and your company to legal action or bad public relations. Negative comments about your company or its employees undermine your own recruitment efforts. Who would want to work there after hearing your critical remarks?

Successful recruiting involves more than just knowing where the best employees are found, but this information will save valuable time and money when it is time to fill a position.

## Hiring

Risk management procedures should be followed in the hiring process. If a human resources department is available, consult them. If not, consult with an attorney before beginning. Check company policy carefully and follow it to the letter. What you say, ask, or don't ask during screening or interviewing can be a matter for legal action. In general, you may not ask about or make hiring decisions based upon age, race, religion, ethnic group, physical appearance, handicaps, or family matters (such as marital status or numbers of children). If you are not clear on the specific requirements, find out before you do anything or talk to any prospective employees. Be sure that any forms you use, such as employment applications, have been reviewed and are legally acceptable. Any notes you take during screening calls or interviews may be made public, so be careful with your comments. Even if you don't write something down but make a statement indicating your hiring decision was influenced by age, race, religion, or other taboo area, it may also become public knowledge. Be equitable and unbiased in your staffing decisions.

The Americans with Disabilities Act (ADA), enacted in 1992, can significantly impact the hiring process. The language of the statute is not specific, and much of its interpretation will depend on the outcome of pending and future litigation (cases in court). Under the ADA, many conditions are considered disabilities. In the past, small businesses were exempt from some state and federal laws applying to business and this may still be the case with some provisions of the ADA. Consult with an attorney familiar with the ADA for specifics. Presently, it appears that businesses must bear the cost of making any accommodations necessary to hire the disabled, with the maximum expenditure not clearly established. This means that if a qualified disabled person applies for a job you are filling, your business must make any structural changes to the office or purchase any special equipment required to enable the disabled person to perform the job.

**DECIDE WHAT YOU WANT**
This is not an easy step, but doing it well, before you do anything else, will save time and trouble. A job description may be necessary for the position you are filling. If one exists already, review it carefully to be sure it still applies and, if possible, discuss it with the person who is leaving the job. Make any modifications that are necessary to keep the job description up to date. Parts 2 and 3 of this book discuss more specific job descriptions for employees most likely to be found in oral healthcare delivery. If this position is new or there is no existing job description, write one. This will require group input, from anyone reporting to, working with, or supervising the person in the job being described.

After you have a good job description, write a brief description of the person who might best fill that position. Don't be too narrow in your focus—remember that the person who is just right may not be exactly what you expect. A job description might state that the person will be required to answer the phone, even how

many phone lines. The job description will not say, however, that the person needs
to have a clear speaking voice and a friendly attitude. If these attributes are important to your business, put this in your notes about who might best fill the position.
Be careful not to be discriminating. For example, do not rule out the hearing-
impaired for the reception job. It is quite possible that a hearing-impaired person,
with the aid of proper electronic equipment, could perform this task well. The
ADA may require that the company provide such equipment.

Finally, define the minimum acceptable requirements, the qualifications that
are advantageous but not mandatory, and any additional skills or experience that
would be useful. Having this description will simplify the rest of the process.

**ADVERTISE**
Advertise if you must. If you and your managers have been maintaining recruitment functions, you might not have to advertise. Just spread the word through
your various networks that you have a position open and qualified candidates
should start calling. Since some companies and many government agencies
require that all job openings be advertised, be sure to comply with these rules if
they exist. This will not prevent anyone you have found through your own recruitment efforts from applying as well.

Where to advertise and what to say in the ad will be determined by budget and
by the position you are filling. Before you begin, determine your budget for
recruitment and hiring, including not only advertising but also possible travel
expenses to interview out-of-town applicants. More than one ad may be necessary,
so don't invest the entire advertising budget on the first one. Advertising costs vary
considerably depending on the publication. Choosing the best place to advertise
will depend on the position you are trying to fill.

The purpose of advertising is to inform as many *qualified* people as possible that
you are hiring. Employment ads can be found in local, regional, or national newspapers; specialty, trade, or professional journals; or job registries, to name a few.
Employment advertising isn't limited to print media, either. You can recruit from
schools and colleges through their placement offices or by posting notices. Cable
television and radio also run help wanted ads. The secret to cost-effective employment ads is reaching qualified candidates.

To illustrate, if hiring a secretary, you will probably advertise in local or regional
(city) papers. Since most businesses require secretaries or clerical personnel of
some type at one time or another, there are usually numbers of them available in
most job markets and you need not go to highly specialized publications to reach
them. Since this is not a highly paid position, you probably would not be willing to
pay travel expenses for candidates to come in for interviews or relocation expenses
if you did find someone from out of town. For this reason, you will not need to
advertise at the national level. There are, of course, exceptions to this. If you are in
an out-of-the-way location or the job market for secretaries is highly competitive in
your area, you may need to look further afield to find the right person.

On the other hand, if you want to hire a physician with experience treating
radiation sickness, you will have to get the message out nationally, and probably
internationally as well. If active in this field, you probably already know all the
qualified individuals through your networking activities and so advertising will not

be necessary. If you are the hospital administrator, however, advertising might be necessary. You would not advertise in the newspapers of the world's 50 largest cities because the costs would be considerable and the chances slim that a qualified individual would happen across your ad. Your advertising money would be more wisely spent by placing ads in professional journals for physicians. For a job this specialized, you might be more successful with an ad in a journal that focuses specifically on issues related to cancer therapy or bone marrow transplants than in a widely read journal, such as the *Journal of the American Medical Association.* You only need to reach maybe five or ten people in the whole world. Even if they aren't looking for a job change, they will probably know anyone qualified who is.

Experience with something as rare as radiation sickness is very particular. Contacts within the professional community might be more successful than advertising in such a case. The point is to be specific. If you have to advertise, put your ads where they are most likely to be read (or seen or heard) by the person you want to hire.

What should you say in an employment ad? As much or as little as necessary to attract qualified applicants. Be sure to state as much as possible about any requirements that are inflexible. For example, if a bachelor's degree is the minimum education acceptable, that is, you will not even be willing to interview or cannot hire anyone without a bachelor's degree, state the requirement in the ad. There is no point in having to screen out 40 unqualified callers when putting a few words in the ad could eliminate them ahead of time. On the other hand, if a degree is preferred but not required, you may not want to say this in the ad, for it might discourage that one person who is perfect for the job from calling just because he or she lacks a degree. Along with stating any specific requirements for employment, your ad should, if at all possible, make the job and the company sound as attractive as possible. You want qualified individuals to want to work for you.

## SCREENING

Screening can be done by mail or phone, depending on your personnel resources and timetable. The purpose of recruitment activities, including advertising, is to encourage people looking for a job to contact you, or you may contact someone you know who is qualified. The purpose of screening is to reduce the number of applicants to those few who meet your minimum requirements and seem likely to be right for the job. Interviewing is a time-consuming and therefore expensive process. Your screening procedure should eliminate all candidates who do not meet your requirements but not exclude those who might be right. It is at this stage that your work on the job description and position requirements will begin to pay off.

Who should do the initial screening? If time is sufficient to receive resumes and review them in advance, the person making the hiring decision may have time to screen the mail. If you advertise and the initial screening will be by phone, you may be receiving a lot of calls. Will the person(s) making the hiring decision have time to take all the calls? Whoever takes the screening calls will have to be available to talk on the phone throughout the day for however long the ads run.

Whether it is you, the manager, or someone else who does the screening, there are a few points to keep in mind. First and most importantly, don't forget the legal obligations, as discussed under Risk Management. Generally, you may not ask any personal questions or about an applicant's criminal record, age, family plans, or other obligations. What is said or asked during a screening call may be the subject of legal action. Second, preparation and training are necessary. Have a list of questions prepared in advance, even if you will be doing the screening yourself. In this way, you can be sure that you have gathered all the necessary information and that the caller meets your minimum requirements. Get the names and phone numbers of all callers, even those you decide not to interview, in case you reconsider and want to contact them for an interview later. Finally, use the screening call to make interview appointments. This means that if someone else is doing the screening, that person will need to know the schedule of the person who will be doing the first interview.

## INTERVIEWS

How many interviews an applicant has will depend on your company and the position being filled. Some applicants need only be screened, by mail or phone, and interviewed once before being hired. The more skill a job requires and the more critical it is to the business, the longer the interview process will take. The purpose of interviewing job applicants is to be sure they meet your requirements and to assess their "fit" for the job. A certain degree of subjective decision making is involved in the hiring process, but making the process as objective as possible reduces the risk of hiring the wrong person.

Determining qualifications was the first step in the hiring process. You can now use the job description and qualifications you've chosen to assess the candidates objectively. The screening process should have eliminated the unqualified applicants. Interviewees should at least meet your minimum requirements and possess additional skills and qualifications to make them likely candidates. At the first interview, you may conduct additional skills tests, for example, have typists take a typing test or programmers write a computer program. You cannot legally give job applicants any type of personality profile tests, such as the Briggs/Myers test. Although you may give some performance-related tests, such as typing tests, all candidates must take the same test under the same conditions.

Interviewing is an art. A good interviewer does more than ask the right questions. Some people may be good at it naturally, but most learn by experience. This is a good reason to include more than one person in the interview process, even if only as observers, and it will be valuable training for future managers (so you can promote from within). Some of the subjective information to be gathered during the interview process is how well the prospective employee will fit in with the rest of the company. Be careful, though, that you don't make all employees fit the same mold, for there can be great strength in diversity. Innovative ideas, fresh attitudes, and new methods can be valuable assets. Don't rule someone out just because he is different.

Get input from the same people you consulted about the job description—supervisors, co-workers, subordinates—those who will work with the person you hire. The new employee will be assimilated more smoothly if co-workers feel they were involved in the hiring decision. If more than one person will be interviewing the candidates, or you will be working in groups, agree in advance how you will proceed. That is, decide who will ask questions, take notes, and so on. If inexperienced people are involved, review the risk management procedures with them and have them begin as observers only.

## REFERENCES

Don't skip this step, as is common practice. Get references, business and personal, for all applicants whom you are seriously considering. Since you are hiring the person for business, your most reliable source of information will be business references, especially previous employers. If the applicant is young or inexperienced, you may have only personal references. Also check the applicant's educational background and any other pertinent information supplied on the resume or employment application.

Look for gaps in the employment record. If someone has been unemployed for a period of months or years, find out why. If the person is not what he claims, it is best to find out before offering him a job.

As with all other aspects of employment, references may also present a legal problem. All the principles of risk management apply to giving employment references. The less said about an ex-employee, the better, even if the person left on amicable terms. For this reason, some companies refuse to give references or will only confirm dates of employment and possibly salary or reason for leaving. You may have to request reference information on a letterhead, in writing. If you encounter this kind of resistance when checking references, don't assume that the applicant has something to hide. You may just be encountering another company's risk management procedures.

Your company should also have a policy regarding employment references. Limit the information you will release to confirming dates of employment and salary. These should be brief, not detailed, statements, giving only the date the person started work at your company and the date the person left. Confirm the ex-employee's salary only if that person has given the information to the new company. Reference requests should be made to you in writing, on a letterhead. You never know who is on the other end of a phone call. Putting everything in writing doesn't eliminate all legal risks, but it will reduce them and give your firm a written record of what has transpired.

## EMPLOYMENT CONTRACTS

When you decide to hire, you will make an offer of employment. You can do this on the phone, but it is best to follow up with a letter.

Job applicants should see a copy of the job description early on in the interviewing process, for it is difficult to tell from an ad or brief description what a job really entails. In this way, you will avoid wasting a good deal of time interviewing individuals who, in the end, realize that your job is not for them. By the time you get to the job offer, the prospective employee should have a firm idea what the job will involve and what your company is like. In the interview process you will be selling your job to the applicants as much as they are selling their services to you. When you find the perfect person and offer him a job, you want eager acceptance.

After the job offer is tendered, you may enter into contract negotiations with the applicant, if not already begun during the interview process. The contract may be very short or quite complicated, depending on the job opening. Always seek legal advice on the contract, before you sign it, no matter how simple it appears. Some specific examples of employment contracts for oral healthcare providers are included in Parts 2 and 3.

## Termination

Everything that has been said previously about risk management applies doubly to job termination. Ex-employees have little motivation to protect your company. Employees may choose to leave (voluntary termination) for any variety reasons. Or they may be laid off (placed on indefinite leave without pay) or fired (forced termination).

### UNEMPLOYMENT INSURANCE

Every employer pays unemployment insurance to the state in which the business is located to fund benefits to the unemployed. The company's unemployment insurance contribution is a portion of the employees' earnings and can vary from a fraction of 1% to 7% or more. For example, if an employee earns a total of $900 in one pay period and the employer's unemployment insurance rate is .3%, the employer pays the state $27. This can add up to a significant amount of money. For example, if a small business with about eight employees has a monthly payroll of $45,000 and an unemployment insurance rate of 6%, the company will owe the state $2700 per month. Normally, unemployment compensation is capped, meaning that employers are obligated to pay insurance only up to a certain percentage of salary.

Why is this discussion included under Termination? The employer's unemployment insurance rate is determined by how many ex-employees file for unemployment benefits and how many employees it has. The actual amounts vary from state to state, but a minimum level applies to all employers, even those who have never had an unemployment claim against them. Each time an ex-employee files for unemployment (makes an unemployment claim), the company's insurance rate may be adjusted upward. A company that has had many unemployment claims will have to pay a very high rate of unemployment insurance.

Any unemployed person can file for unemployment, but not all will receive payment. Again, the rules vary from state to state. Be aware of the laws that affect your location, for your employer's insurance rate is affected only by claims that are paid. Who can file for unemployment payments? An employee who quits, who is laid off, or who is fired—basically anyone, for any reason. Whether the claim is paid depends on the actual case, and you can probably find at least one example of a case being paid for just about every reason. In short, it is difficult to predict accurately which claims will be paid and which won't. Strive to keep your unemployment insurance rate as low as possible. Legal advice from someone experienced in your area may be helpful.

### VOLUNTARY TERMINATION

When an employee gives you notice (tells you he is quitting), you can accept this decision, negotiate about how long he will work before leaving, or negotiate to keep him on. If you have subtly encouraged him to move on, let him go as quickly as possible. If he is a great resource to the company, try to find out why he is leaving. In either case, act quickly. Nothing is gained from keeping a "short timer" hanging around. Evaluate what his work is really worth to your business and determine whether there are points you can bargain on to keep him with you. You don't want to offer him more than he's worth, but you don't want to lose a valued employee if you can avoid it.

## FORCED TERMINATION

Firing is difficult and painful for everyone involved. For the person being fired, this may mean significant changes in life-style or lower self-esteem. For the manager doing the firing, it often comes at the end of months of work toward motivating and improving the employee's performance. It may be that termination was a decision forced on the manager by pressure from higher levels of management or from clients. When making a decision on firing or preparing to give the employee notice, try to be sensitive to the emotional elements involved so that the situation does not get out of control.

Essentially, any employee-at-will, or one working without a contract, can be fired for any or no reason. Contract employees, by contrast, have termination clauses in their contracts. You are not required to give an employee-at-will a reason for termination, but it should be clear to you. Be fair and unbiased in your decision making. Hiring and firing come with high price tags, in both dollars and stress.

There are different views on how to handle the termination interview. It may involve a lengthy discussion and review of all the employee's performance evaluations. Keep in mind the legal risks. Anything that you say may be the basis of a lawsuit. Remember that it is not necessary to give any details about the decision, although you may feel that this approach is best within your company or in a specific situation.

In today's litigious society, the "fast fire" has become very popular. The fast fire begins with a very short (five minutes or less) termination interview, then the employee is required to leave as quickly as possible. Someone should accompany the fired person from the time of the termination interview until he leaves the building. This will not only give him some support at a difficult time, it will prevent acts of theft or sabotage. The fast fire can save emotional wear and tear on both the employee and the employer.

Whether you choose the short or long termination interview, be clear that the objective is to fire the employee and do not be persuaded otherwise. Do not be moved by emotional pleas, as this will not correct a significant problem the employee has or change the situation if layoffs are necessary.

Almost everyone is surprised to be fired, even when repeatedly warned that it would happen. The employee will probably be upset. Plan for this. For example, if possible, conduct the interview in the employee's office, rather than in your office, so that he can compose himself privately. This will also make it easier for you to end the interview, by returning to your own office. If you hold the termination interview in your office, you may have a distraught employee in there for a long time. Consider the time of day and day of the week, if possible, and minimize the time the fired employee has to complain to other employees.

Take precautions regarding security and technology in advance. You know when the termination interview will take place. Alert building security, if it exists. Make arrangements to have the employee turn in his keys or to have the locks changed. Be sure that all valuable computer data are safely backed up and safe from a disgruntled employee's sabotage. Make arrangements to have the person escorted from the office. This will make it easier for the person than having to leave alone, especially if the employee has boxes of personal effects. It will also be the responsibility of the escort to see that the employee does not leave with any company property.

Be prepared to discuss the firing with remaining staff members. Know what you will say and when. For example, hold a special staff meeting for this purpose if a regular meeting is not scheduled shortly after the termination. The other employees will have questions and be worried. Depending on the conditions of the termination or your agreement with the ex-employee, you may not be able to discuss specifics of the case, but be honest and as factual as possible. Be careful not to slander or make the ex-employee a scapegoat.

Job security is a significant concern for most people. Having regular evaluation systems in place can help employees to assess their own performance, make improvements if necessary, or strengthen a case for a raise or advancement.

## Temporary Help

Staffing is a dynamic process. Even in a stable firm, people may be coming and going from various positions at different times. Staff members may be on vacation or sick leave. For many positions, temporary help is available. Temporary placement agencies now offer services for clerical, secretarial, reception, bookkeeping, accounting (including CPAs), labor, electronics assembly, nursing, medicine, dentistry, and dental hygiene, to name a few. If staff changes or fluctuations leave you short-handed, consider hiring temporary help from an agency. The costs of such staffing range from 10% to 60% of the temporary employee's wage. There are also costs associated with not hiring help when you need it. Direct costs include lost sales and decreased production. The indirect costs include loss of client goodwill, poor service, and decreased production in another area partially dependent on the output of the missing employee. When making a decision about hiring temporary help, be sure to consider what it may cost directly and indirectly not to have help.

As with other staffing areas, it helps to be prepared, especially if your employees are highly specialized. Different agencies specialize in different types of employees. Become familiar with the services offered in your area, and the quality of different agencies, before you need to call them in an emergency.

## Associated Costs

There are costs associated with staffing changes. They include the costs of losing an employee, such as higher unemployment insurance rates or decreased production; the costs of hiring a new employee, such as placement fees and training; and the costs of taking up the slack created by an unfilled position, such as hiring temporaries. Any of these costs can be substantial. For these reasons, staff turnover should be kept to a minimum. It is often more cost effective to keep on an employee whose performance is minimally acceptable than to hire someone new.

Let's consider a worst case example, where everything possible goes wrong. We will discuss a receptionist position, one that does not require extensive education or in-office training, in a high-tech electronics firm. The receptionist comes to work with a gun and is immediately fired for violating company policy against having weapons on company property. It is Monday morning. The phones are ringing. Customers and field sales representatives are calling in. There was no cross-training for the receptionist position and the one other person who understands how to operate the phone system is out on maternity leave, so no one in the building can even get calls, let alone messages. What is this mess going to cost?

You have to hire a temp immediately. The only available agency charges you an outrageous price for the temp, and you have to have an emergency service call from the company that services your phone system to train the temp. You lose two big sales because angry customers couldn't get through. Your best sales rep is out looking for other employment opportunities because he's not getting good support. The ex-receptionist files for and receives unemployment benefits and your unemployment insurance rate goes up 2%. You miss a critical deadline trying to sort out the receptionist mess and therefore may not be eligible for a raise. You don't have any contacts to recruit a new receptionist, so you have to advertise, for five weeks, before finding a qualified candidate.

Meanwhile, you're still paying for a temporary receptionist, who still doesn't quite understand the phone system and isn't always polite to customers. You spend so much time on the phone screening job applicants and interviewing that you miss another important deadline. In the end, you hire the least objectionable candidate because he seems better than the temp. The new receptionist spends a month learning the phone system and the rest of his responsibilities. He loses four phone messages for the company president and hangs up on your biggest client before you realize that he must go. You fire him. He applies for and receives unemployment benefits. Your rate goes up yet again.

You've exhausted all your sources for receptionists and hire a replacement through an agency. You now incur a placement fee equal to 20% of the receptionist's annual salary. The (second) new receptionist now has to go through four weeks of training before he's really up to speed, and so on. Imagine what the scenario would have been like if this situation involved an employee with specialized education, years of experience with the company, and critical understanding of the industry!

The point is that staff turnover is expensive. Hire the best people you can and do your best to keep them. This doesn't mean that you have to keep employees who aren't performing or that you have to go to any lengths to keep the acceptable employees. It does mean that you have to go out of your way to reward the best and make your company an attractive place to work.

## Performance Evaluation

Don't treat your employees like children. If you have more than two or three, they will quickly drive you crazy. Hire the best staff you can and give them training and room for development and advancement. Establish a regular system of objective setting and performance evaluation, and involve each employee in setting personal objectives and preparing performance evaluations. Employees dependent only on their manager for evaluation may not be very productive. People need to evaluate their performances on a daily, ongoing basis, or errors may be caught too late to correct or a wonderful innovation may go unnoticed. Clear objectives and periodic reviews are crucial for good performance.

Performance evaluation can be a valuable motivational tool if used correctly. Evaluation begins with strategic planning (see Chapter 1) by involving employees in the plan's development. As action plans are developed, responsibilities for specific tasks or actions will be assigned to groups or individuals and can be a basis for developing performance evaluation objectives. In this way, you can be sure that employees will be evaluated on items for which they are specifically responsible. Also, you can be sure that all employees are working in accordance with the overall strategic plan. Some employees may have general or ongoing responsibilities in addition to their responsibilities for specific action plans. In developing the performance evaluation mechanisms for these employees, be sure to set objectives and define actions for these areas of additional responsibility.

It is not important what you call the individual performance objectives. Call them goals, objectives, or actions, or whatever suits the situation. You may want to use the same terms you use for organizational planning, so that individuals have long-range goals, short-term objectives, and specific action items.

Performance evaluation (PE) objectives for individuals should include an observable action, a measurable result, and a deadline for accomplishment. You will notice that these are essentially the same elements you included in the organizational objectives. One employee may have just a few PE objectives or many, depending on the nature and scope of the person's responsibilities. Each PE objective should include all three elements—action, result, and deadline.

The action in the PE objective must be observable, or you will not be able to use it for evaluation. For example, *complete, write,* and *assemble* are observable actions, whereas *motivate, change attitude,* and *be willing* are not. If it is the employee's responsibility to motivate others, the observable actions are the things the "others" do that can be observed, such as increased sales volume.

Suppose you want the employee to be willing to pitch in and help the customer service department. If you write the PE objective "to be willing," what happens when, at the time of the evaluation, the employee says, "I was willing," but you think he wasn't? You will be stuck in an endless argument over the employee's willingness, with neither side able to offer any proof to substantiate its claims. If you write the objective to state "Answer the phones in the customer service department whenever requested to do so by the department head," you will have a mechanism to follow up. If the department head never made a request, this item is not significant. If the department head made four requests, and the employee refused each one, then you have a point of substandard performance.

Each objective should have a measurable result. For example, *a completed training manual, 100 patients treated,* and *5% increase in sales* are measurable results. *Treat patients, increase revenues,* and *produce newsletters* are also observable results, but are too vague to be measured with any degree of objectivity. The objective should be more specific; for example, *treat 100 patients per month, increase revenues by 20%, produce four quarterly newsletters* are statements that can be used for PE. The objective should state exactly what level of performance is expected.

Each objective should include a reasonable deadline or state that the objective relates to an area of ongoing responsibility. The deadline should be specific, such as July 4, end of the third quarter, or one week before the conference begins. Whenever possible, the employee should be included in setting the deadlines, so that he is working on a timeline that he feels he can meet. On the other hand, if the employee can't meet the deadlines imposed by the demands of the position, such as client requests, either he should not be in that position or other factors are influencing the situation that you need to investigate.

Keep in mind that the reason for writing PE objectives is to use them in performance evaluation. All of the employee's responsibilities should be covered by specific objectives. Whenever possible, have the employee prepare the performance evaluation, as part of getting the job done, to document who, what, when, where, how, and why the PE objectives were or were not met. It is much more efficient to have the employee perform the task of documenting things as they happen, rather than have a manager try to find the information weeks or months after a project is complete. The outcome of the performance evaluation should not come as a total surprise to the employee. An employee who has been working toward personal objectives and documenting that work all along will have self-evaluated and know what to expect, good or bad.

Frequent evaluations are more effective than infrequent evaluations, although you do have to limit the amount of time spent on evaluation or you won't have time to get any work done. Frequent evaluations will allow you to spot and correct performance problems before they get out of hand and will allow you to reward outstanding performance in a timely manner. The exact schedule for performance evaluation will vary from job to job and, often, within a job, depending on the work load. More specifics on oral health delivery are discussed in Parts 2 and 3.

During the evaluation, it should only be necessary to go through the objectives and review whether each was met, with the expected result, and within deadline. For unmet objectives, uncover the cause and include new objectives for correcting the problem or improving the employee's performance. Acknowledge and praise employees for meeting their objectives, or they may think it's not really important that they have. Commend and reward employees who perform beyond expectations so that they will be motivated to continue to do so. Positive reinforcement works faster and lasts longer than negative reinforcement. Keep criticism focused, and use it only when necessary. Foster a commitment to quality within your organization by applauding good performance whenever it occurs.

## Summary

Human resources are people. They are part—the most important part—of all the resources with which a manager has to work. Those who work most successfully with people are often leaders as well. Managing human resources requires that you always be concerned with risk management. If people present one of the most challenging and rewarding aspects of management, they potentially represent some of the worst disasters. A good manager, like a good scout, is always prepared for staffing changes—hiring, firing, and evaluation. A good manager also has to work with planning and with people to see that everyone is moving in the same direction at an appropriate pace.

## Review Questions

1. List at least three reasons to follow policies and procedures consistently.

2. If you are currently employed, look at the policy or procedure manual at your office. If not, obtain one for your school or volunteer organization. Are any of the policies out of date? If so, why? Are new policies needed? In what areas?

3. Write a new policy for one of the areas identified in Question 2.

4. Which of the following represent risk management issues—situations in which the manager in charge may need to consult company risk management policy or may require legal advice?

    a. Taking calls from job applicants calling about a help wanted ad

    b. Firing one of your employees

    c. Talking to your neighbor about how your secretary is always late for work

    d. a and b only

    e. All of the above

5. What is the manager's role in recruitment? In hiring? In termination?

6. Write a job description for a job that you have held.

7. Which of the following are costs associated with staff turnover?

    a. Advertising

    b. Placement fees

    c. Staff training

    d. a and c only

    e. All of the above

8. Name five other costs associated with staff turnover.

9. List the three components to include in performance evaluation objectives.

10. Write a performance evaluation objective for a job you have held.

## SUGGESTED READING

Basset, L. C., & Metzger, N. (1986). *Achieving excellence: A prescription for healthcare managers.* Rockville: Aspen Publishers.

Blanchard, K., & Johnson, S. (1982). *The one minute manager.* New York: William Morrow & Co.

Cohen, W. A. (1990). *The art of the leader.* New Jersey: Prentice-Hall.

Naisbitt, J., & Aburdene, P. (1985). *Re-inventing the corporation.* New York: Warner Books.

Peters, T. (1987). *Thriving on chaos.* New York: Alfred A. Knopf.

Peters, T. J., & Waterman, R. H. (1982). *In search of excellence.* New York: Warner Books.

Who's excellent now? (1984). *Business Week,* November 5.

## REFERENCES

Carnegie, D. (1981). *How to win friends and influence people.* New York: Simon and Schuster, p. 46.

Kotter, J. P. (1990). What leaders really do. *Harvard Business Review,* 68(1): 103–111.

# Chapter 3

# Finance

## Objectives

After reading this chapter and completing the review questions, the reader should be able to:

- Describe the time value of money.
- Define the meanings of the line items of a balance sheet.
- Define the meanings of the line items of an income statement.
- Define the meanings of the line items of a cash flow statement.
- State the importance of cash flow to a business.

After reading this chapter and completing the review questions, you will not be a financial expert or accountant, for the methods for actually preparing financial statements are beyond the scope of this text. Certainly many managers, especially in small business, do prepare or direct the preparation of financial statements. It does require additional training for which courses and books are available, if this is one of your managerial responsibilities. For the purposes of this book, we will assume that the financial statements are prepared by an accountant who is available for consultation and that your role as a manager will be to interpret the financial statements. Preparing the statements is merely a process; extracting and understanding the business's condition based on the numbers presented is one of the crucial arts of business management.

## THE TIME VALUE OF MONEY

It is obvious that money is valuable stuff. By definition, money equals value. A 100-dollar bill would be just a piece of paper without the backing of the federal government. Money has time value because it costs money to borrow money. If you don't have it when you need it, you will have to pay to borrow what you need. The longer you keep the borrowed money, the more you will have to pay in interest, hence the term "time value." For example, money that is in *your* account, versus somewhere else, could be earning interest for *you*, instead of for the person or corporation whose account the money *is* in when you don't have it.

In an inflationary period, money left sitting idle or payments not collected cost both interest and inflation. For example, if a client pays you $100 by check and you leave the check in your in box for a month before depositing it, you have lost interest payments, which at 12%, could have amounted to $1 for the month. During a period of inflation, the $100 may have less purchasing power one month later than when you received it. If inflation is at 1% that month, this amounts to another $1.

Okay, so $2 doesn't amount to much. It might cost you that in gas to drive to the bank to deposit the check. But a business collects more than $100. Suppose it was $10,000. Left in a drawer for a month, as in the first example, the business would lose approximately $200, which might be a significant portion of the month's profit. Suppose the bookkeeper made this a regular habit, and each month left checks totaling $10,000 sitting idle for four weeks before depositing them. In a year, the business would have lost $2400 in unearned interest and decreased purchasing power.

An often unrecognized cost of unused money is opportunity cost. The unused or uncollected money could be doing some important work *right now*. If you don't have the funds available at the right time, you may miss a valuable investment or business opportunity. Cash, the most liquid asset of any business, should be working for you at all times.

## FINANCIAL STATEMENTS

What are financial statements and what do they tell you? The most common set of financial statements you will encounter are the balance sheet, the income statement, and the cash flow statement. Together, they represent a snapshot of a company's financial status at the moment they were prepared. Consider them the company's financial "vital signs." Although they will not tell you everything there is to know about the company's total corporate well-being, they will give you some important clues. For this reason, you, as a manager, should be able to interpret the "big picture" represented by the financial statements.

Although Part 1 has dealt with many types of businesses as examples, finances can be very industry specific. For this reason, this chapter will deal with the Smallville Dental Group, P.A. as an example of financial statements. P.A. indicates a corporate structure often used by healthcare practices and that the Smallville Group is a professional association. In some states, this structure may also be called a professional corporation (P.C.). This structure is similar to a corporation, usually indicated by Inc. Being a P.A. gives the practice legal status as a corporate body and gives the owners some protection from liability. For example, if the P.A. is sued, it is the corporation that is sued, not the owners directly (although this often follows).

All businesses will probably use the three basic financial statements—the balance sheet, the income statement, and the cash flow statement—but there will be significant differences in the magnitude of numbers presented and in exactly what they represent. All three statements are presented together.

## Footnotes

Always read the footnotes included with every financial statement. Footnotes are important. They explain how the accountant arrived at the amounts stated. As you will see in the following discussion, there are different ways of valuing many of the items and the footnotes give the details of the methods used to prepare a particular statement. You need to check the footnotes attached to the financial statements in order to understand what the numbers on the financial statement actually represent.

## Fiscal Calendar

Fiscal year and fiscal quarter are terms used frequently in financial discussions. The fiscal year does not have to begin on January 1 and end on December 31 and so may differ from the calendar year. Although it is possible to change a company's fiscal year, it is seldom done (check the footnotes attached to the financial statements) and the Internal Revenue Service (IRS) strictly limits the number of such changes. A corporation's fiscal year will begin and end at the same time each year. For example, the federal government begins its fiscal year on October 1 and ends it on September 30.

Finances may be summarized on a weekly, monthly, or quarterly basis. A financial quarter is three months (1/4 of the year) and will vary according the corporation's fiscal year. For example, if the company begins its fiscal year January 1, and ends it December 31, the first quarter will run January 1 through March 31; the second quarter, April 1 through June 30; the third quarter, July 1 through September 30; and the fourth quarter, October 1 through December 31. For the federal government, the first quarter runs October 1 through December 31; the second quarter, January 1 through March 31; the third quarter, April 1 through June 30; and the fourth quarter, July 1 through September 30.

While there are many reports, financial and otherwise, that a manager will need to use, it is always a good idea to carefully review the quarterly and yearly financial statements to check the corporation's vital signs.

## The Balance Sheet

Refer to Figure 3.1, the balance sheet of the Smallville Dental Group for 1996. The balance sheet may also be called the statement of financial condition or the statement of financial position.

The Smallville Group's fiscal year ends on December 31. The figures shown on this balance sheet are the amounts in the various accounts as of midnight, December 31, 1996, when the group "closed its books" for the year. This is probably not how the numbers looked on regular business days immediately before and after

| Current Assets | | Current Liabilities | |
|---|---|---|---|
| Cash | $ 35,000 | Accounts Payable | $ 7,000 |
| Accounts Receivable | $ 25,000 | Operating Expenses | $ 22,000 |
| Inventory | $ 2,000 | Income Tax Payable | $ 4,000 |
| Prepaid Expenses | $ 10,000 | Short-Term Notes Payable | $ 0 |
| Total Current Assets | $ 72,000 | Total Current Liabilities | $ 33,000 |
| | | Long-Term Notes Payable | $180,000 |
| **Property, Plant, & Equipment** | | | |
| Equipment & Furniture | $240,000 | **Total Liabilities** | $213,000 |
| Accumulated Depreciation | $ 34,000 | | |
| | $206,000 | **Stockholders' Equity** | |
| | | Common Stock | $ 20,000 |
| | | Dividends to stockholders | $ 0 |
| | | Retained Earnings | $ 45,000 |
| | | | $ 65,000 |
| | | **Total Liabilities** | |
| **Total Assets** | $278,000 | **& Stockholders' Equity** | $278,000 |

**Figure 3.1**    *Balance sheet, 12 months ending December 31, 1996, Smallville Dental Group, P.A.*

December 31, but unless something unethical was going on, there should not be significant differences over a short period.

Notice that the balance sheet is divided into two columns. The one on the left (Current Assets), gives the details of the company's assets; the right-hand column (Current Liabilities) itemizes the company's liabilities. Assets are the pluses, things that add value to the corporation. Liabilities are the minuses, things that decrease the value of the corporation.

Each line of the balance sheet represents an account. Asset accounts generally are Cash, Accounts Receivable, Inventory, Prepaid Expenses, Equipment & Furniture, and Accumulated Depreciation. The liability accounts typically are Accounts Payable, Operating Expenses, Income Tax Payable, Notes Payable, Capital Stock, and Retained Earnings. The accounts don't actually exist as separate bank accounts, but are considered separately so that the use of funds is easier to follow. Firms may vary the accounts used to tailor the information presented to their particular needs.

## ASSETS

*Current Assets*   Current Assets are the short-term (one year or less), more-liquid (easily turned into cash) assets of the Smallville Group.

***Cash***   The Cash account is the amount of cash on hand or in bank accounts. Cash refers to money that is liquid, easily accessible, and not involved in long-term investments.

Cash balances for a dental practice may vary seasonally because patient flow tends to vary this way. You could expect to see low cash balances around December, when payments are notoriously slow, and higher cash balances in spring and fall. Watch for trends. If the first and third quarter cash balances are usually high and suddenly a third quarter report shows a very low cash balance, the situation bears some looking into. If a year-end cash balance is unusually low compared to other years, slow collections or other financial weakness may be indicated.

Excess cash that has been invested will be listed separately under Marketable Securities, a line that does not appear on the Smallville balance sheet. Marketable securities include such investment vehicles as government bonds or notes, stocks, bonds, or mutual funds. If this account is used, it usually appears right after cash.

***Accounts Receivable***   Accounts receivable are moneys due to the corporation but not yet collected (received). For a dental practice, receivables are usually generated from clients who did not pay at the time services were rendered or from cases awaiting insurance payments. A high accounts receivable balance would probably indicate collection or billing problems. Keep accounts receivable as low as possible, so that this cash can accumulate interest or pay the company's bills, not remain in the clients' or insurance companies' accounts.

***Inventory***   Products waiting to be sold are the inventory. In a service business, such as oral healthcare delivery, only a small portion of the company's assets will be tied up in inventory, since the product is treatment time, not hardware. A dental hygiene practice may have some inventory if it sells products like home care devices or fluoride for home use. An orthodontic practice might have inventory in the form of braces and appliances.

Inventory levels should be kept as low as possible, because unused items sitting on the shelves are not earning the company any money and tie up cash. On the other hand, if inventory levels fall too low, slow delivery and lost customers may become a problem for the company. The goal is to get the inventory just in time to turn it around and sell it (or use it in a manufacturing process).

***Prepaid Expenses***   Prepaid expenses are expenses paid in advance. Items included in this account might include insurance premiums, rent deposits, and property taxes.

***Other Current Assets***   The other current assets accounts that may be used include Notes Receivable and Other. Notes receivable are amounts due to the company within the year. Other is, of course, the catch-all category. Prepaid expenses may be included in the Other account instead of listed separately.

***Total Current Assets***   The line below the amount in the prepaid expenses account indicates that the lines above are totaled. The total of cash, accounts receivable, inventory, and prepaid expenses is listed as Total Current Assets.

***Property, Plant, & Equipment***   The second category of the Smallville Group's assets is called Property, Plant, & Equipment. This category might also be titled Noncurrent Assets.

***Equipment & Furniture***   The Smallville Group does not own the land or building where the office is located, so they do not have any property (land) or plant (building) assets. They do have furniture and equipment. For a dental practice, the investment in equipment can be considerable. Equipment valued in this account would be substantial items, expected to last more than one year, and is commonly referred to as capital equipment. Other types of equipment, like disposable prophy angles, would be considered supplies. These assets are listed at their purchase price, not their replacement value (which may be considerably different). Another term used for this category is Fixed Assets.

***Accumulated Depreciation***   Fixed assets, although long-lasting, do eventually wear out. For this reason, they are depreciated (devalued) over time. Check the footnotes attached to the financial statements, because the IRS accepts several methods of depreciation. You will notice in Figure 3.1 that the amount of accumulated depreciation is subtracted from the value of the equipment and furniture to derive its current value to the corporation at the time the balance sheet was prepared.

***Other Assets***   Other Assets is an account that may appear under Property, Plant, & Equipment. Other assets may include long-term investments, real estate, or intangibles. Investments that will generate income a year or more after the date of the financial statement are included as other assets. Short-term debts due the corporation would be considered with Accounts Receivable or other current assets. If the business owns real estate, land, or buildings not used by the business, they would be considered with other assets.

   The intangible assets account may include patents, copyrights, or trademarks owned by the business. Healthcare practices do have an important intangible asset: goodwill. Goodwill is a term used to describe the faith the clients have in a practice and its healthcare providers. Its value is its ability to keep clients returning to the practice and referring others. It is a difficult thing to value, but it is a significant asset because the client base is equal to goodwill. Without the clients, the practice won't generate any income. The value of goodwill becomes an issue when a practice is being sold and the practitioners for whom the clients hold the goodwill are leaving the practice.

***Total Assets***   The last line in the assets column is Total Assets. This represents all of the Smallville Group's assets, both current and long term.

## LIABILITIES

***Current Liabilities***   The right-hand column lists the liabilities, beginning with Current Liabilities. These are the obligations the corporation must pay within the year.

***Accounts Payable***   Accounts payable are the unpaid invoices (bills) the practice owes it suppliers. It is helpful to compare this number to the accounts receivable.

If payables are higher than receivables, you must wonder how the business will manage to pay its debts (see Ratios on pp. 55–57). Although this situation sometimes occurs, it bears investigation. For a dental practice, a consistent pattern would indicate the business may be running in a deficit (loss) situation, depending on the other assets of the corporation.

Note that the accounts payable of one business represent the accounts receivable of another. For example, if Smallville owes a dental lab $4000, this amount is an account payable for Smallville and a $4000 account receivable for the lab. Keep these terms straight when calling or writing to inquire about your payables and receivables. If calling about your bill with the lab (your accounts payable), you want to talk to someone in the lab's accounts receivable department.

Most major suppliers grant credit to other businesses, so purchasers need not pay cash on delivery (COD). Most credit terms require that invoices be paid within 30 days, although this figure is often negotiable.

Many companies offer a discount for early payment. A common policy is "2% ten," meaning a 2% discount is given if the invoice is paid within 10 days of receipt. Although it is wise to offer such a discount, as many firms do take advantage of it, it is not a good idea to take the 2% ten discount. The reason relates back to the time value of money. Keep your money as long as possible, even longer than 30 days if you can. The money will do you more good than it will do your supplier. Of course, there is more involved in this issue than just paying bills. You don't want to ruin your relationship with a good supplier over a late payment.

Inventory that you have received but not yet paid for is included with accounts payable. At the same time, the asset account Inventory is increased by the value of the goods received. For a business where inventory management is critical, inventory might be listed as a separate account under Accounts Payable.

*Operating Expenses*    Operating expenses may include rent, payroll taxes (income tax goes in a separate account), utilities, insurance (general liability, malpractice), and bad debt, among others.

*Income Tax Payable*    Income tax payable is the tax on the amount of income the business has earned since its last tax payment but that is not yet due to be paid. Income tax payments are due quarterly and yearly. Payroll taxes, including income tax withheld for employees, is an operating expense.

*Short-Term Notes Payable*    Short-term notes payable are loans due within one year. These may be due to a bank (usually), an individual, or another corporation. Many dental practices do not engage in short-term borrowing, but it is very common in other industries. For example, a company that manufactures autoclaves must purchase the parts to assemble the autoclave well in advance of being able to sell it. This creates a cash flow problem for the manufacturer who must come up with the money to pay for the parts long before collecting the money for the finished product. It is often necessary to borrow, from a bank, for 60 to 90 days, or for whatever the cycle from manufacturing to sales is, to cover the cost of in-house inventory.

***Total Current Liabilities***   The line below Short-Term Notes Payable indicates that the preceding lines are summed to arrive at the total current liabilities, which are due within a year.

***Long-Term Notes Payable***   Long-Term Notes Payable lists loans due more than one year from the date the balance sheet was prepared. Many dental practices begin with little capitalization because newly graduated dental students don't have cash to start a practice. To afford the needed capital equipment (dental chairs, etc.), they borrow the capital from a bank on terms longer than one year, often 5 to 30 years. Shorter loan periods are more common, although all such loans may be increasingly hard to come by.

***Long-Term Liabilities***   Long-term notes payable are listed under Long-Term Liabilities. There may be other long-term liability accounts, such as Deferred Credit, Rent, or Other. Deferred credit is work for which a client has paid but that has not yet been done. The work is still "owed." Rent may be included if the lease includes amortization of a special build-out. This is common for dental practices, since they usually require special changes to the interior architecture to run plumbing and air and gas lines. The charge for these modifications is often spread out (amortized) over the entire period of the lease. The Other long-term liabilities may include mortgage loans or bonds.

***Total Liabilities***   Total Liabilities represents all of the corporation's short-term (current) and long-term debt obligations.

***Stockholders' Equity***   Stockholders' Equity may also be called net worth or net assets. It is what the business owes the owners after all other obligations are paid. It may include a number of accounts. The Smallville Group is a professional association, a corporate entity. If it were a proprietorship, owned by one person, or a partnership, owned by more than one person, but not incorporated, it would not have stockholders and this category would then be called net worth or net assets. For a proprietorship or partnership, the net worth amount would represent the amount originally invested by the owners, plus any additional investments they made when they gave the practice more money, plus the accumulated profit.

A corporation issues stock, so Smallville has a stock account. There are different types of stock issues, such as common, premium, or discount, and, depending on which had been used, these would be listed as separate accounts. Stock is sold to raise money to capitalize, or finance, a business.

***Common Stock***   Common stock represents all issued or unissued shares of stock. It represents shares of equity in the business. This is what the owners of the practice got when they invested money in the practice. State laws govern who may invest in a professional association. For example, most require that the owners of a dental practice must be dentists.

***Retained Earnings***   Retained earnings are profits allowed to remain in the business. The account may also be called Retained Surplus. Stockholders are often paid dividends—meaning they make money on their investments—which are paid from retained earnings, reducing the amount of retained earnings. You will see that Smallville did not pay any dividends in 1996, nor did it issue any new stock. The line below Retained Earnings indicates that the lines above (Capital Stock and Retained Earnings) were summed to get the total of stockholders' equity.

Another format dental practices commonly use for this section lists the starting balance of retained earnings at the beginning of the period, the current earnings for the period, nondeductible expenses, and dividends paid. See Figure 3.2 for an example.

The dentist-owners of the Smallville Group are taking most of their money in salary, as employees of the P.A. In sole proprietorships or partnerships, the dentist-owners may not take a salary but instead take the profit of the practice as their income. Income taken as salary is a tax-deductible expense for the practice (an operating expense) and the dentists pay tax on the money only once, as part of their personal income. Whatever current earnings remain in the practice are taxed at the corporate rate which, in Maryland for example, is 34%. Smallville has therefore tried to reduce the taxable income of the practice by having the owners take most of their money in salary. If dividends are paid out of retained earnings, those stockholders receiving the dividends will pay personal income tax on them. In this way, the money is taxed twice: once as corporate profit and once as personal income.

The Smallville Group paid $22,100 in taxes on the current earnings, and the stockholders received a total of $50,000 in dividends. If each stockholder paid 28% personal income tax on the dividends received, they would have paid a total of $14,000 in taxes. The total taxes paid by the practice and the dentists would have been $36,100. If, on the other hand, the dentists had taken all of the current earnings as salary ($65,000) and each had paid 28% personal income tax on it, the practice would not have had any current earnings, would not have owed any taxes, and would not have paid any dividends or taxes. The total amount of tax paid would have been $18,200.

Retained Earnings is the line that balances the balance sheet. After total liabilities are subtracted from total assets, what remains is profit (retained earnings). Total assets always equal the total liabilities plus the stockholders' equity:

Total assets = total liabilities + stockholders' equity.

It is important to remember that retained earnings represent a paper profit. For the owners of a company to actually receive the retained earnings, all of the

| | |
|---|---|
| Retained Earnings as of 12/31/95 | $45,000 |
| Current Earnings | $65,000 |
| Nondeductible Expenses | $22,100 |
| Dividends to Stockholders | $50,000 |
| Retained Earnings as of 12/31/96 | $37,900 |

**Figure 3.2** *Alternative method for reporting retained earnings*

company's assets would have to be sold off and all of its bills would have to be paid. This is the definition of liquidating a company. Furthermore, the stockholders would receive only the exact amount listed as retained earnings if all the estimates used to prepare the balance sheet were exactly correct and if all the assets could be sold for the values given on the balance sheet. There are also substantial costs associated with liquidation, and these would have to be deducted from retained earnings as well. In short, the owners of the Smallville Dental Group, P.A. would not get much cash, if any.

## The Income Statement

Refer to Figure 3.3, the income statement for the Smallville Dental Group. The income statement may also be called the earnings statement, the statement of operations, or the profit and loss (P&L) statement. The income statement is a summary of the revenues (sales) and expenses for the period (in this case, one year).

*Income from Services*   The top line, Income from Services, is the total amount received, or expected to be received, from sales or services. It may also be referred to as Sales Revenue, Gross Sales or Gross Income. It does not include sales tax collected, but does include accounts receivable.

   The lines that follow, through Income Tax Expense, are deducted from Income from Services to calculate the "bottom line," Net Income (discussed later).

*Operating Expenses*   The operating expenses account may contain many different items, including salaries, benefits, legal fees, and supplies. It may contain all the business's operating costs except cost of goods sold, depreciation, and income tax. Often, other accounts listed are under Operating Expenses, such as General, Marketing, or Administrative. Smallville has broken this down into Salaries, Lab Fees, and Indirect Costs (such as administrative costs). They might also have used just

| | |
|---|---|
| Income from Services | $663,000 |
| Operating Expenses | |
| Salaries | $409,000 |
| Lab Fees | $ 15,273 |
| Indirect Costs | $115,230 |
| | $539,503 |
| Operating Earnings | $123,497 |
| Depreciation Expense | $ 34,000 |
| Interest Expense | $ 21,600 |
| Earnings Before Income Tax | $ 67,897 |
| Income Tax Expense | $ 22,897 |
| Net Income | $ 45,000 |

**Figure 3.3**   *Income statement, 12 months ending December 31, 1996, Smallville Dental Group, P.A.*

two headings, Direct Expenses, such as providers' salaries and lab fees, and Indirect Expenses (which would include other salaries).

The income statement for a manufacturing business would probably have an account for cost of goods sold. This account would include the cost to the business of buying the products it resold or parts it used to manufacture the things it did sell.

Cost of goods sold is related to inventory (and inventory that is part of the accounts payable liability). Some, probably most, of the goods sold will be gone. Those that remain in-house at the time the financial statement was prepared, in this case, midnight, December 31, 1996, are accounted for under inventory.

Some businesses use a Gross Margin account. Gross margin is equal to the sales revenue minus the cost of goods sold. Since dental practices are service businesses selling expert time, most of the expenses show up under operating expenses because this is where salaries go. A manufacturing business, on the other hand, may spend significantly more on cost of goods sold, because it has to purchase products materials or parts before reselling them. Its manufacturing process may, or may not be, labor intensive.

***Operating Earnings***   Operating Earnings is what is left after subtracting Operating Expenses from Income from Services. In the case of a manufacturing business that lists Gross Margin, Operating Earnings is equal to Gross Margin minus Operating Expenses.

***Depreciation Expense***   As mentioned previously, fixed assets, such as buildings or equipment, are devalued, or depreciated over time. Every year, each of these capital purchases becomes worth less, and this decrease in assets must be accounted for. That is the purpose of the Depreciation account. Depreciation is not an actual cash expense (no money has left the practice), but eventually the equipment will wear out and be worth $0.

***Interest Expense***   Interest expenses can be significant and so are usually listed separately from other operating expenses.

***Earnings Before Income Tax***   Earnings Before Income Tax is what is left after deducting Operating Expenses, Depreciation Expense, and Interest Expense from the Operating Earnings. This is roughly the amount the practice will pay income tax on.

***Income Tax Expense***   Income tax expense is the amount of income tax the business pays. Payroll taxes for employees are included with operating expenses.

***Net Income***   As mentioned previously, this is the bottom line, what remains after all possible expenditures have been deducted from revenue. Although it is certainly a significant number, it does not tell the entire financial story of the business. It is important to watch trends, analyze the other financial statements, and compute the ratios (discussed later) to understand the true financial status of the company.

## The Cash Flow Statement

Two methods can be used for financial reporting: the cash basis and the accrual basis, used by the Smallville Group. There are important distinctions between the two. You should be familiar with both methods, as they are both used.

Refer to Figure 3.4. The following discussion covers the line-by-line descriptions of the cash flow statement presented. Remember that the Smallville Group uses the accrual method of accounting and that this cash flow statement is in the indirect format.

*Cash Flows from Operating Activities*   The first section of the cash flow statement relates to operating activities. When reading the statement, remember that numbers in parentheses are negative.

*Net Income*   Net income is the amount from the bottom line of the income statement. It is the income remaining after all possible expenses have been deducted.

*Accounts Receivable*   In this case, there has been an increase in accounts receivable. This does not represent positive cash flow because this money has not yet been collected.

### Cash Flows from Operating Activities

| | |
|---|---:|
| Net Income | $45,000 |
| Accounts Receivable | ($25,000) |
| Inventory | ($ 2,000) |
| Prepaid Expenses | ($10,000) |
| Depreciation Expense | $34,000 |
| Accounts Payable | $ 7,000 |
| Income Tax Payable | $ 2,200 |
| | $51,200 |

### Cash Flows from Investing Activities

| | |
|---|---:|
| Purchases of property, plant, & equipment | ($ 5,000) |

### Cash Flows from Financing Activities

| | |
|---|---:|
| Short-Term Borrowing | $      0 |
| Long-Term Borrowing | $      0 |
| Common Stock Issue | $      0 |
| Cash Dividends to Stockholders | $      0 |
| **Net Increase in Cash During Year** | $46,200 |

**Figure 3.4**   *Cash flow statement, 12 months ending December 31, 1996, Smallville Dental Group, P.A.*

*Inventory*   This account also appears on the balance sheet. It represents in-house inventory that has been paid for but has not yet been resold. The inventory that has been sold appears on the income statement in the Cost of Goods Sold account. The Inventory account represents negative cash flow because this is an expense.

*Prepaid Expenses*   These are the expenses for which the company has paid in advance, such as insurance. This account represents negative cash flow because this is an expense.

*Depreciation Expense*   As the value of property, plant, and equipment decreases, so does the company's net worth. This "loss" must be accounted for. This is the purpose of the Depreciation expense account. Note that depreciation does not involve any actual cash expenditure and therefore is not negative on the cash flow statement.

*Accounts Payable*   This account represents invoices that the company has received but has not yet paid. Accounts payable represent positive cash flow because the company has received these assets as goods or services but has not yet had to pay for them.

*Income Tax Payable*   This is the amount the company owes in income taxes but is not yet due; therefore it is not yet negative cash flow. The line under this amount indicates that the figures above have been summed to yield the total of all cash flows from operating activities.

*Cash Flows from Investing Activities—Purchases of Property, Plant, & Equipment*   In this case, the Smallville Dental Group purchased $5000 worth of new capital equipment. This was an expense, but it increased the company's net worth by the value of the equipment. In the following years, as the equipment is devalued to $0, this amount will be decreased under Depreciation expense.

*Cash Flows from Financing Activities*   This section gives the details of how the company raised capital during the year.

*Short-Term Borrowing*   The Short-Term Borrowing account would include any bank loans or notes payable that are due within one year.

*Long-Term Borrowing*   The long-term borrowing account would include any bank loans or notes payable that are due in more than one year.

*Common Stock Issue*   A corporation could raise more capital by selling stock. There would be a separate account for each type of stock issued.

*Cash Dividends to Stockholders*   If dividends were paid to stockholders, this amount would be reported in this section.

*Net Increase in Cash During Year*   The last line is the total of cash flows from operating activities, cash flows from investing activities, and cash flows from financing activities. If a company has had a decrease in cash during the period (this value is in parentheses), it is important to determine why.

## DIFFERENCES BETWEEN ACCRUAL BASIS AND CASH BASIS ACCOUNTING

In *cash basis* accounting, expenses and income are reported when they occur, in other words, when money actually changes hands. For example, a client visits your office in June and pays her bill that day. The income is recorded for June. If, however, the client doesn't pay the day of her visit (when the income was earned), but waits for a bill to be sent at the end of the month, and the payment isn't received until July, the income is recorded in July, when the payment is received. In cash basis accounting, expenses are handled the same way. If you receive a shipment in September, with an invoice for net 30 payment (the payment is due 30 days later), the expense is included in October, when you pay the invoice, not in September, when the invoice is received.

Using the *accrual method*, income and expenses are reported when they are incurred, not when they are collected or paid. In the preceding examples, when the client visits your office in June, the income is recorded in June, whether or not she pays the bill at that time. The invoice received in September is recorded as an expense in September, not in October, when the invoice is paid.

The difference in accounting methods affects the figures on the financial statements. Using the cash basis method, accounts payable and accounts receivable would not appear, because these events haven't happened on the books yet. The payables appear when they are paid, and the receivables appear when they are collected. A business doing most of its buying and/or selling on credit would probably not use cash basis accounting because this would not give a clear representation of the company's finances. As in the case of the fiscal year, it is possible to shift from one accounting method to another, but the IRS strictly limits if, when, and how often such shifts may occur.

You can see in Figure 3.4 that the Smallville Dental Group uses the accrual basis. Its cash flow statement is presented in the indirect format. Figure 3.5 is an example of the Smallville Group cash flow statement presented in the direct format. The first section, Cash Flows from Operating Activities, is the only one that differs from Figure 3.4.

*Cash Receipts from Services*   This account contains the amounts for net income and inventory. It does not contain accounts receivable. A manufacturing company might call this account Cash Receipts from Sales.

*Cash Payments for Operating Expenses*   This account includes all the cash that the practice has actually spent during the period to finance its operating activities (including salaries). It does not include accounts payable. A manufacturing business might also have a separate account for cash payments for products.

The Cash Payments for Interest and Cash Payments for Income Tax accounts do not include accrued interest or taxes not yet paid. Note that there is no depreciation account on a direct format cash flow statement because this money is never actually spent.

**Cash Flows from Operating Activities**

| | |
|---|---|
| Cash Receipts from Services | $638,000 |
| Cash Payments for Operating Expenses | ($552,767) |
| Cash Payments for Interest | ($ 19,600) |
| Cash Payments for Income Tax | ($ 14,433) |
| | $ 51,200 |

**Cash Flows from Investing Activities**

| | |
|---|---|
| Purchases of property, plant, & equipment | ($ 5,000) |

**Cash Flows from Financing Activities**

| | |
|---|---|
| Short-Term Borrowing | $ 0 |
| Long-Term Borrowing | $ 0 |
| Common Stock Issue | $ 0 |
| Cash Dividends to Stockholders | $ 0 |
| **Net Increase in Cash During Year** | $ 46,200 |

**Figure 3.5**   *DIRECT method cash flow statement, 12 months ending December 31, 1996, Smallville Dental Group, P.A.*

The cash flow statement for a company using the cash basis would use the direct format. The Financial Accounting Standards Board accepts both formats, so you may see a company operating on the accrual basis using the direct format for the cash flow statement. It is up to the company's management (or outside board of directors) to choose the methods that best meet the needs of the company.

The financial statements can also be used for projection. For example, when reviewing a third quarter report, you may be able to extrapolate the data to predict whether there will be an overall decrease in cash for the year. An art and a science are involved in doing financial projections, requiring both additional study and experience. The first step, however, is to understand the information as it is presented in the financial statements.

## MANAGING CASH FLOW

Poor cash flow management will put you out of business faster than any other problem. Without cash on hand to pay critical bills, such as payroll, your business is in serious jeopardy.

Cash flow is the day-to-day exchange of any form of money—checks, cash, electronic transfers, and credit card credits and debits—that is necessary to keep a business alive. You pay bills for materials, salaries, and services; you receive income from clients and other sources. Money for cash flow does not come from loans or investors, though interest payments on loans do come from cash flow. A healthy company has sufficient cash flow to pay all its bills on time. One in trouble constantly scrambles to find extra money here and there to avoid lawsuits for nonpayment. Most small businesses, like dental practices, operate between the two extremes.

Cash flow management is the proactive planning of the use of each receipt and each expenditure. Far too many business react to bills and the income stream, seeming almost surprised by each arriving invoice. Every successful company has a person tasked with anticipating expenditures and income and balancing the two to ensure continued business health and viability.

The objective of cash flow management differs from that of standard accounting practices. Normal accounting is strategic. It is directed primarily at ensuring the business meets the owners' goals and complies with IRS regulations and banking conditions. Cash flow management is tactical in nature, a day-to-day battle to keep the creditors at bay or happy. There are two elements to successful cash flow management:

1. Regular reporting of the business's income and expenditures

2. Ongoing analysis and action planning based on data in the reports.

***Regular Reporting***   An old business maxim states that you should "measure everything." You must measure your business income and bills payable on a weekly basis. Successful management includes creating procedures for regular activities and then ensuring the procedures are followed. Reporting is a critical activity you can easily proceduralize. Make sure the reports are completed on the same day each week (Fridays are logical), so you can plan your schedule around them. The best mechanism is a weekly report that includes the following:

**Current assets:**

Petty cash on hand

Cash in checking

Other cash assets (money market funds, etc.)

Aged accounts receivable, with a detailed listing of each

Backlog and estimate of when each backlogged item will be paid

**Current liabilities:**

Aged accounts payable, with a detailed listing of each

Anticipated new cash needs

(Backlog is work already started or contracted for that can quickly be completed and converted to cash or receivables.)

Though it might seem like a lot of work to generate this information each week, if you build a system to acquire and log the data, the process shouldn't take more than 15–30 minutes per week. For instance, if you use a computerized accounting system, then generating accounts receivable (AR) and accounts payable (AP) statements is no more work than pressing a button. Use a form for the rest of the data and have the front desk personnel fill in the blanks by the close of business each Friday.

Put the most important numbers in a spreadsheet. Fill in one line a week. With time, you'll generate a valuable historical record of the business useful for tracking seasonal patterns. Figure 3.6 is an example of such a spreadsheet.

In Figure 3.6, Current Backlog includes those services you project will be billable in the next 30 days (such as cases you expect to complete). This is near-term, almost cash, practically as good as the real thing. Mod. QR is a modification of the quick ratio (see Ratios, pp. 55–57). The quick ratio is a common measure of business health and is defined as (cash + AR)/(AP). This modification, defined as (cash + AR + current backlog)/(AP), gives a more accurate measure of the real near-liquid current assets liabilities. A ratio lower than 1.00 indicates more short-term liabilities than assets—a deadly situation. In the example in Figure 3.6, the ratio is steadily falling, a warning of impending disaster.

*Analysis and Planning*   With minimal training, anyone can gather and collate raw report data, but the manager must set aside time each week to study the numbers, identify the threats and opportunities, and take action. Opportunities are easy to spot and use. If you have far more cash in checking than payables, move some cash to a high-yield account. Keep enough petty cash on hand for reasonable needs, but not so much that it becomes a desirable target for thieves or so much you are losing a substantial amount by not collecting interest. If the current backlog skyrockets (not likely in clinical practice), you might want to hire temps to quickly convert the potential income into cash.

It's important to identify and fix problems. Effective cash management starts with the aged AR report. Never permit a client to exceed 30 days on a payment without initiating corrective action. A surprisingly high number of businesses do extend credit and then make little determined effort to collect when the bill is due.

Shortly before the bill is 30 days old (or whatever your policy is), call your client and ask whether the service was satisfactory or whether there was a problem. Remind the client that the bill is coming due, then state that you accept credit cards, checks, and cash and that finance charges are applied to overdue balances. After the bill is 30 days old, become more aggressive—politely at first, then with increasing vigor. Never accept defeat at the hands of an answering machine or voice mail. It is possible to contact anyone, given enough determination. Leave messages and follow up within a day. Get promises of payment and then follow up regularly, making the client deliver on the promise. The squeaky wheel gets the grease. Problem clients are often delinquent on many accounts, not just yours. Be annoying enough that they want to pay you, and not the other, less aggressive, creditors.

| | A/R | A/P | Checking | Petty Cash | Other Cash | Current Backlog | Mod. QR |
|---|---|---|---|---|---|---|---|
| 1-8-94 | 45,550 | 55,072 | 15,553 | 105 | 20,000 | 5,112 | 1.57 |
| 1-15-94 | 54,917 | 68,906 | 20,443 | 50 | 20,000 | 4,665 | 1.45 |
| 1-22-94 | 39,474 | 62,194 | 16,324 | 94 | 20,000 | 4,665 | 1.30 |

**Figure 3.6**   *Cash flow weekly snapshot*

Collections can be a sensitive area. Be sure that the person handling it has regular, adequate training to handle the process politely, effectively, and in accordance with office policies. It is a bad marketing move to have providers (dentists and hygienists) or practice owners handle collections, although managers and owners should be available to talk to clients if so requested.

Collecting on receivables can be tedious and boring, but you can never let it drop or give up in frustration. Remember that if you don't contact these people, you may not get paid! Call, keep calling, send dunning letters. Train a staff member to do most of this work, and make it fun. Find someone with the tenacity of a bulldog and a heart of steel who can take the rejection but keep on calling. Complement her on her skills. Make sure she processes income checks so she sees the fruits of her labor.

If an account gets out to 60 or 90 days, pass it on to a collection agency. The longer you wait to do this, the harder it will be for the agency to collect. Collection agencies vary widely in services and expense. Some take 30–50% of the amount collected. Others require a small up-front payment that covers collection on a predefined number of accounts. If you expect to go to collections often, interview a number of collection agencies and select one that meets your needs. Check their references! Pay attention to complaints from clients regarding the methods used by the collection agency.

On the other side of cash flow, never pay a bill early. If the terms are net 30, pay on the thirtieth day or even a little later. Cash is your business's grease. Like an engine, the business will seize without it. Conserve every penny, leaking only when really necessary. Half of cash flow management involves following the precepts outlined here, which can be summed up as "collect early, pay late." The other half is using the reports to project cash needs for a period of several months to come.

Maintain a spreadsheet of all AR and AP, expected near-term backlog, and anticipated bills. List each and every item and the expected due in or paid out date, as illustrated in Figure 3.7. Note that each receivable, payable, and everything currently on order is listed. "Regulars" are those bills that come due each month without fail, like rent and phones. Try to include all expenses and sources of revenues so you can accurately model your cash needs. The second to last line is the total cash required for that week. The last line lists cumulative cash flow—the cash surplus or shortfall, summed across by week. In the example shown in Figure 3.7, income is far short of expenses. Unless action is taken soon, this business may fail.

The data provided by this spreadsheet are invaluable. It can tell whether you can afford a new autoclave or other necessary equipment. A look at your cash flow needs will tell you instantly. If the model projects massive cash needs, you had better start generating more revenues, get a loan or equity financing, or work a deal with creditors to survive.

# RATIOS

Understanding a company's financial position involves more than reading the financial statements. Ratios are one of the tools used most often for financial analysis. Many different ratios are used, and they are roughly divided into three groups: solvency ratios, efficiency ratios, and profitability ratios. Solvency ratios are

|  | July 23 | July 30 | Aug 6 | Aug 13 | Aug 20 | Aug 27 |
|---|---|---|---|---|---|---|
| **A/R** | | | | | | |
| Accardis | 1833 | | | 1833 | | |
| Bennet | | 224 | | | | 1233 |
| Harris | | | 334 | | | |
| Neslab | | | | 5546 | | |
| **Total A/R** | 1833 | 224 | 334 | 7379 | 0 | 1233 |
| **A/P** | | | | | | |
| Payroll | | 18900 | | 18900 | | 18900 |
| Allied | | | 564 | | | |
| Allied | | | 175 | | | |
| AppPlus | 520 | | | | | |
| AT&T | | | | | 138 | |
| Austronics | 91 | | | | | |
| **Total A/P** | 611 | 18900 | 739 | 18900 | 138 | 18900 |
| **On Order** | | | | | | |
| Hall | | | | | | 543 |
| Vantage | | 676 | | | | |
| Franklin | | | 25 | | | |
| **Regulars** | | | | | | |
| Rent | | 4254 | | | | |
| GBS | | 332 | | | | |
| Insurance | | 567 | | | | |
| Phones | | 212 | | | | |
| Utilities | | 446 | | | | |
| Citibank | | 400 | | | | |
| Cash | 611 | 25787 | 764 | 18900 | 138 | 19443 |
| | 1222 | −24341 | −24771 | −36292 | −36430 | −54640 |

**Figure 3.7** *Cash flow spreadsheet*

used to determine a company's ability to meet its financial obligations. Efficiency ratios describe how efficiently the company uses its assets, especially its receivables. Profitability ratios describe the company's performance.

Ratios are calculated by dividing one account or group of accounts by another account or group of accounts. We will discuss only the two most commonly used ratios here: the quick ratio and the current ratio.

The *quick ratio*, also known as the acid test or liquid ratio, measures a company's ability to cover its current liabilities with its current liquid assets (can easily be converted into cash). The formula is

$$\text{Quick ratio} = \frac{\text{cash} + \text{AR}}{\text{current liabilities}} .$$

In the case of the Smallville Group, this would be

$$\frac{\$40,000 + \$60,000}{\$55,400} = 1.80.$$

A ratio of 1.0 or higher is advantageous, indicating that there are sufficient liquid resources to meet the company's financial obligations in the worst case. The usual ratio may vary considerably from industry to industry, depending on the nature of the businesses involved and their financing methods. A quick ratio that falls below 1.0 should be cause for concern and further investigation, unless a lower quick ratio is standard in a particular industry.

The *current ratio* measures a company's short-term debt-paying ability. The formula is

$$\text{Current ratio} = \frac{\text{total current assets}}{\text{total current liabilities}}.$$

In the case of the Smallville Dental Group, this would be

$$\frac{\$136,000}{\$55,400} = 2.45.$$

Investors and banks generally like to see a current ratio of 2. That is, the company has about $2 of assets for every $1 of liabilities.

Both the quick ratio and the current ratio are solvency ratios. They are the most commonly used ratios because they are numbers with which investors and creditors are concerned. Other *solvency ratios* include current liabilities to net worth, current liabilities to inventory, total liabilities to net worth, and fixed assets to net worth.

Investors will also be concerned with *profitability ratios*, such as the following: return on sales (ROS), return on assets (ROA), and return on net worth (RON). Investors want to know that their money is going into a profitable venture.

$$\text{ROS} = \frac{\text{net profit after taxes}}{\text{net sales}}$$

$$\text{ROA} = \frac{\text{net profit after taxes}}{\text{total assets}}$$

$$\text{RON} = \frac{\text{net profit after taxes}}{\text{net worth}}$$

Managers often use *efficiency ratios*, such as the following: collection period, sales to inventory, assets to sales, accounts payable to sales, and sales to net working capital. Managers use these ratios to monitor and adjust operational efficiency.

$$\text{Collection period} = \frac{\text{AR / sales}}{\text{365 days}}$$

$$\text{Sales to inventory } = \frac{\text{net sales}}{\text{inventory}}$$

$$\text{Assets to sales } = \frac{\text{total assets}}{\text{net sales}}$$

$$\text{Accounts payable to sales } = \frac{\text{AP}}{\text{net sales}}$$

$$\text{Sales to net working capital } = \frac{\text{net sale}}{\text{net working capital}}$$

A final ratio, one commonly discussed though not used in private dental practice, is the price/earnings (P/E) ratio. This ratio is calculated for companies that are publicly held. The first step is to calculate the earnings per share (EPS):

$$\text{EPS } = \frac{\text{net income for year}}{\text{total number of stock shares}} .$$

The P/E ratio equals the current market price per stock share divided by the earnings per share:

$$\text{Price/earnings ratio } = \frac{\text{current market price per stock share}}{\text{earnings per share}} .$$

Publicly held corporations must report their earnings per share as part of the income statement. Private corporations, which includes most dental practices, do not use the EPS or P/E ratio because their stock is not traded. The owners would use one or all of the profitability ratios to judge the value of their investments. The P/E ratio is often mentioned when people are discussing their investments in the stock market.

### Summary

Financial statements, ratios, and some aspects of money management, including the time value of money and managing cash flow, have been briefly covered. Financial management techniques specific to oral healthcare delivery are discussed in Chapter 8.
   Managing finance is, in some way, a part of most managerial jobs. The nuances of financial management are industry specific, but some concepts are common to all types of business. Reading and understanding financial statements and the ratios derived from them is a basic managerial skill. Not all managers need to be experts, but for them financial numeracy, like verbal literacy, is vital for effective management.

## *Review Questions*

1. Change the Smallville balance sheet (Figure 3.1) so that the Cash account contains $45,000, and recalculate the other accounts, as necessary, to rebalance the assets and liabilities.

2. Change the Smallville income statement (Figure 3.3) so that Operating Earnings equals $32,000, and recalculate the "bottom line."

3. Change the Smallville cash flow statement (Figure 3.4) so that the Depreciation Expense equals $30,000 and recalculate the Net Increase in Cash During the Year, changing other accounts as needed.

4. Suppose that the Smallville Group borrowed $50,000 with a 10-year bank note to equip a new operatory. Rewrite the financial statements to reflect this change. Note that in this case the depreciation expense will not change because the new equipment will not begin to depreciate until the following year. Also, for this example, the $50,000 will completely cover the cost of buying and installing the new equipment, so that accounts payable will not be affected. The new operatory will not be operational until January 2, 1997.

5. The financial statements of publicly traded companies are available to interested investors. Obtain the financial statements for a company you are interested in. Many large companies in the healthcare industry, for example, corporations that own hospitals, are publicly traded.

6. Using the financial statements obtained in Question 5, calculate the quick ratio and the current ratio for the company you have selected.

7. Is the company you selected in Question 5 a good investment opportunity? Calculate its P/E ratio. (*Hint:* Check the *Wall Street Journal.*)

8. If possible, obtain the financial statements either for a business at which you are or have been employed or for your college or university. Review these statements and record any insights you have gained about the operations of the business of which you have been a part.

## SUGGESTED READING

Gumpert, D. E. (1990). *How to really create a successful business plan.* Boston: Inc. Publishing.

Livingstone, J. L. (Ed.) (1992). *The portable MBA in finance and accounting.* New York: John Wiley & Sons.

Simini, J. P. (1990). *Balance sheet basics for non-financial managers.* New York: John Wiley & Sons.

Tracy, J. A. (1989). *How to read a financial report.* New York: John Wiley & Sons.

# CHAPTER 4

# Marketing

•————————————————————————————————•

## *Objectives*

After reading this chapter and completing the review questions, the reader should be able to:

- Define marketing.
- Define the three P's of marketing.
- Define public relations.
- Define advertising.
- Define sales.
- Describe the purpose of marketing management.

•————————————————————————————————•

This chapter discusses marketing management and the three main components of marketing: public relations, sales, and advertising. Like planning, human resource management, and finance, marketing is a complex field. Imparting a complete understanding of the subject is beyond the scope of one text. This chapter will familiarize you with the basic concepts, so that you will have a foundation for understanding marketing management specific to oral healthcare delivery as discussed in Parts 2 and 3.

## WHAT IS MARKETING?

Every author and management guru has a definition of marketing. They range in length. David Ogilvy (1983) says that he once heard marketing defined as "objectivity." David Gumpert (Ogilvy, 1983) defines marketing as "identifying your customer prospects and determining how best to reach them." Robert Davis (1990) combines the definition of marketing with a description of the role of the marketing manager:

> Marketing describes a business function, like production, finance, research—or marketing. These functions are the key organizational components of any company. Marketing's essential responsibility is to create customers—just as production creates products. The marketing executive, in this role, employs an assortment of marketing variables to craft an effective marketing strategy.

Each of these definitions has merit, but considering the three together gives more depth to the meaning. Objectivity is important. Marketing is often considered a creative function, but without objectivity, it may be an ineffective function. Identifying customers, reaching them with your message, and getting them to use your product or services are the central objectives of marketing. Marketing should do more than create customers; it should drive the creation of products. The best way to launch a successful new product or service is to find a need and fill it, not to invent something neat and then try to find a way to sell it.

What is the purpose of marketing management? Coordinating the marketing variables to develop a successful marketing strategy. Marketing strategy is often discussed in terms of the three P's—position, price, and promotion.

## Position

The position of a product or service is described in terms of its market segment. Once you have described the market segment, or the target audience for the product or service, you have described its position. Many products or services are aimed at more than one segment. This approach may even be a key to successfully marketing some products. If you can narrowly define your market segments, all of your marketing activities can be designed to appeal to a specific group. This approach will increase the chances of your product or service being accepted by a particular segment.

One product may be used in entirely different ways by different market segments. Existing product lines can be given new life by finding a new use, or market segment, for them. For example, take a product as simple as the paper cup. Paper cups appeal to different groups of customers for different reasons. Fast-food restaurants purchase cups that are eye catching and upbeat to make the beverage seem appetizing. Paper cups used with water coolers, however, don't need this graphic appeal. Paper cups used in hospitals for dispensing medications will have different dimensions and coating requirements. There are many other markets for paper cups and probably quite a few that haven't even been thought of yet. The point is that even though the product remains the same, it may have to be positioned differently for each market segment.

## Promotion

*Promotion* ranges from advertising to public relations to sales presentations. Promotions can be events in themselves, such as concerts sponsored by radio stations. Other types of promotions include "buy one get one free" or "receive a free gift with a purchase," and new types of promotions appear almost every day. Promotions may need to be different for different market segments. Some promotions, advertising, or public relations campaigns can successfully continue unchanged for long periods and some are only effective for a short time.

Promotion can make or break a product or service. For example, actor Bruce Willis was a successful spokesman in making Seagrams Wine Coolers appealing to a young, party-oriented market segment. When Willis was arrested for public drunkenness, however, sales dropped sharply and Seagrams received a lot of public criticism. Willis no longer fit the image with which many young, health-conscious consumers wanted to be associated, and Seagrams, a huge producer of all types of alcoholic beverages, could not afford to be associated with negative effects of alcohol consumption. The problem with the spokesman for the wine coolers also affected Seagrams' other brands. The promotion was having a negative effect on sales and Willis was fired.

## Price

Choosing the right price for a product or service involves a lot more than just looking at what it costs to produce it. Price is an important determinant of position. It tells the customer something about the product or service, whether it is aimed at the discount market, with little luxury or support, or at the upscale market, with a lot of support and individualized attention, or somewhere in between.

A classic example of the effects of price is the Loreal brand of hair color. Originally introduced as a low-cost brand, Loreal did not fair well among the well-established competitors in that market. Without any change whatsoever, the product was repositioned as an upscale, luxury brand by raising the price. It has been promoted with phrases like "because you're worth it" and has dominated its market niche since it moved into the higher-price category.

The Loreal brand also serves as a good example of the connection among the three P's. The product was repositioned by raising its price, which moved it into a new market segment. It was promoted differently, as well: high-profile actress and model Cybill Shepherd became a spokeswoman for the brand in commercials emphasizing its luxury aspects.

Marketing activities include public relations, sales and advertising, the product or service mix, price and position, and, most importantly, the market—the customers. Do not overlook the significance of customers, clients, patients, consumers, or whatever a particular industry calls them. In a highly competitive market, the most successful product or service will the one that best meets the consumers' needs, not necessarily the product or service with the highest quality. What counts the most is consumers' perception that they are getting what they want—value.

A marketing strategy can employ activities in public relations (PR), sales, and advertising, singly, or in any combination (see Figure 4.1). The strategy you select will depend on your industry, product, and budget. For example, soft drink manufacturers, who are competing in a very broad consumer market, must devote a considerable portion of their marketing strategy to advertising. Car dealers must dedicate a large portion of their marketing strategy to supporting sales. Health-care providers in private practice, on the other hand, are often discouraged from

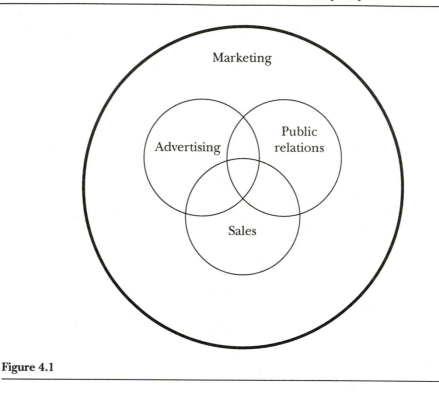

**Figure 4.1**

advertising, do not have any direct sales activities, and must rely almost entirely on public relations.

   Bear in mind that there is no distinct line between the marketing activities of PR, advertising, and sales. They are closely related, and you may find that what begins as a PR program actually involves elements of advertising or that what begins as a sales promotion, supported by advertising, generates a lot of PR.

## PUBLIC RELATIONS

Public relations is not paid advertising, direct selling, or promotional gimmicks, although it has sometimes been associated with all three. Public relations activities can generate advertising, sales, media reports, and public awareness. A public relations campaign is rarely directed at "the public" as a whole, but is usually targeted at a specific segment. Robert Dilenschneider (1990), a well-known public relations adviser, defines PR as "the power triangle," using "communication, recognition, and influence" to advance the agenda.

   Public relations objectives are accomplished through many avenues. Various forms of communication are used, often with or through the press, both broadcast (TV and radio) and print (newspapers and magazines). A primary tool of PR is the press release. Press releases are prepared news items that have traditionally been printed, though video press releases are becoming more common. Press releases are prepared by organizations (or their media advisers) to inform the press of newsworthy events. The information in the press release may be used for the story, or the press release may prompt more inquiry from the media, leading to more in-depth coverage or investigation.

Press releases generally follow a standard format: They are typed, double spaced, on letterhead. Refer to Figure 4.2 for an example of a press release. Note the name and phone number of the contact person is listed prominently at the top, as is the date of the press release. Some press releases are for immediate release. Others are actually sent out in advance, in which case the release date is given instead of "for immediate release." If the press release is longer than one page, the word "—more—" should appear at the bottom of each page. The last page usually ends with "###."

When preparing press releases, keep your company's overall strategic plan and marketing plan in mind. Restrict press releases that you initiate to items that further your organizational goals. There may be times, however, when you will have to issue statements or press releases in the event of a crisis or unfortunate incident. Again, keep your mission in mind.

Consider the following example of public relations in action. On July 17, 1981, a suspended walkway in the Kansas City Hyatt Hotel collapsed, killing 114 and injuring hundreds more. In *Power and Influence*, Dilenschneider (1990), the PR counsel for Hyatt, describes how he handled the incident. He emphasizes that quick action, compassion, and honesty were the keys to successfully managing Hyatt's PR and maintaining a positive focus on solving problems. There were four main points of the plan. In the face of considerable human loss, Jay Pritzker, the chief executive officer (CEO) of Hyatt, *demonstrated compassion* by being constantly available to meet with the families of the dead and injured. Pritzker chartered planes to fly in the loved ones of victims to *help victim's families come to terms with the tragedy.* Hyatt *used money constructively.* Rather than stonewall and hide from any possible implication of fault, Pritzker endowed a fund for the benefit of the families of people who had died and underwrote the cost of psychological help for the survivors. Dilenschneider reports that there was, incidentally, no negative impact from doing this. The fourth point was that Pritzker kept *reinforcing relief efforts* by aiding and commending the officials and public services involved.

We can look back on this incident many years later and see how Hyatt Hotels have faired as a result of this PR effort. Hyatt has done well. There was no explosion of public outrage against the hotel chain, and it was able to manage the lawsuits. People are continuing to use the Hyatt hotels, and Hyatt has even been able to maintain its reputation for architectural innovation (it was found not to be at fault in the structural failure). What could have happened? What if the Hyatt people had not demonstrated openness, honesty, and compassion, but instead had jumped in and tried to just cover all of Hyatt's liability concerns? Hotels are a very public business. A general boycott of Hyatt's facilities could have severely damaged the company financially or even put it out of business. Rancor from the media could have kept the spotlight on the disaster for years.

Dilenschneider uses the Three Mile Island incident as an example of PR gone wrong. In 1979 there was a minor radiation leak inside the Three Mile Island nuclear power plant in Pennsylvania. Partially to prevent panic, the company officials in charge did not begin with openness, honesty, and compassion. Although

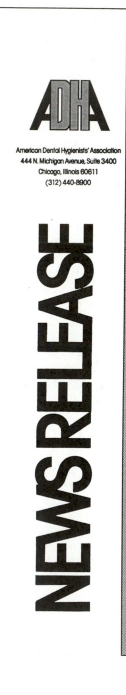

American Dental Hygienists' Association
444 N. Michigan Avenue, Suite 3400
Chicago, Illinois 60611
(312) 440-8900

**Contact:**    Sammie Sumlin              **Date:**  July 27, 1992
**Phone:**      312/440-8900              **For Immediate Release**

**Dental Hygienists Adopt Position to Safeguard Patients**

**Chicago**--After evaluating concerns that attempt to link the transmission of infectious diseases to oral care procedures, the American Dental Hygienists' Association (ADHA) has issued a revised version of its 1991 position statement outlining safeguards for patients and dental hygienists.

ADHA has always emphasized that dental hygienists provide services in an environment of frequent and continual exposure to infectious organisms. And, in order to protect patients and practitioners, the association advocates adherence to universal infection/exposure control precautions and hepatitis B immunization for all dental hygiene students and licensed dental hygienists. In addition, the association has revised its statement to reflect that it recognizes the Occupational Safety and Health Administration (OSHA) standards relating to workplace safety and training. OSHA issued its final rule governing employers' obligations concerning occupational exposure to hepatitis B virus (HBV), human immunodeficiency virus (HIV), and other bloodborne pathogens in March 1992.

Deborah Bailey McFall, RDH, BS, ADHA president, points out that "current scientific and epidemiologic evidence indicates that there is little risk of

-more-

**Figure 4.2** *Press release (Courtesy ADHA)*

**Hygienists Adopt Position**
**To Safeguard Patients**
**Page . . . . 2**

transmission of infectious diseases during oral healthcare treatment
for patients or practitioners if universal precautions are routinely
followed."

The previous statement also called for research that quantifiably
assesses the potential for HIV transmission prior to the formulation
of any public policy regarding testing or potential practice
restrictions. The new statement has been revised to include the
association's opposition to mandatory HIV testing.

The statement also reiterates that ADHA believes dental hygienists
are ethically and legally responsible to provide dental hygiene care
to all patients regardless of their health status.

McFall concludes that "because dental hygienists have direct
contact with blood and saliva from patients who may be infected with
HIV and other viruses, we recognize the importance of taking
necessary precautions to protect patients and dental hygienists while
providing quality oral healthcare."

The Chicago-based American Dental Hygienists' Association is the
largest national organization representing the professional interests
of the almost 100,000 registered dental hygienists (RDHs) nationwide.
The RDH designation assures patients that the dental hygienist has
completed a nationally accredited dental hygiene education program and
is a licensed oral healthcare provider.

--30--

**Figure 4.2** *Continued*

no one was injured as a result of this incident, such a public hue and cry resulted that the entire nuclear power industry was brought to a virtual halt. While there were certainly other factors that brought this about, Three Mile Island was the beginning of the end.

Another example of effective public relations in a crisis occurred in 1982 in Chicago, when over-the-counter acetaminophen (Tylenol) capsules were laced with cyanide. Seven people died. At that time, Tylenol, a product of the McNeil Consumer Products division of Johnson and Johnson, Inc., was the leading over-the-counter analgesic on the market, by a large margin. When the poisonings were discovered, McNeil immediately responded (with openness, honesty, and compassion) and recalled all Tylenol that could possibly have been affected. This was the beginning of a costly process, which continued over many years. In the end, however, the Tylenol brand was saved and has regained much of its market share. If this incident had been mishandled, McNeil might have lost the Tylenol brand name, which it had spent years and millions of dollars promoting. A negative backlash could also have affected other McNeil and Johnson and Johnson products.

It is easy to look back and evaluate PR in action in times of crisis. Public relations is not to be used only for crisis management, however. It can be an integral part of any marketing plan, though not on such a grand scale as required in the examples given here. Communication, recognition, and influence are part of daily business activity.

Communication takes place on many levels and in many directions. Communication within the company, large or small, up and down the chain of command and laterally, is vital to all functions, as was discussed in Chapters 1 and 2. Internal PR can be as important as external PR. Publicize within your organization all positive outcomes, outstanding achievements, and plans for change. Communication also needs to take place from the company to the outside world and from the outside to within the company. Corporate messages should be specifically targeted to customers, or better yet, to specific groups of customers, to others within your trade or profession, to the media, or to politicians or special interest groups, to name a few. Your PR efforts need to be focused, organized, and part of the overall marketing plan, which should, of course, be driven by the company's strategic plan. Information and feedback need to flow from all these groups, and others, into your organization and it needs to reach the right people within your organization.

In the example of the Hyatt disaster, communication between Hyatt management and the press was easy to identify, but there was also a tremendous amount of communication taking place within the Hyatt organization, to be sure that they were delivering a uniform message, to manage their victim and family assistance efforts, and to provide information and to help the rescue workers. Without these multiple lines of communication, or if one had broken down, the outcome for Hyatt might have been very different. Worse yet, live victims trapped in the wreckage might not have been saved or families might not have been together in time of need.

When you communicate about outstanding performance, you are recognizing individual or group achievement. For example, Pritzker recognized the achievements of rescue services in the Hyatt disaster. Another aspect of PR is ensuring that your firm's accomplishments are recognized. This may take some time, but avoid the temptation to proceed in a flamboyant manner. You might also want to publicize individual successes outside the company, especially those related to community service. Achieving recognition is an important part of building influence. If no one recognizes what you have done, you will not be able to build upon your successes.

Influence is not to be confused with influence pedaling, backroom deals, or manipulation. Using influence need not be an unethical practice. To return to the Hyatt example, Pritzker used his influence as the CEO of a major corporation to encourage relief efforts. McNeil Consumer Products, makers of Tylenol, was active in the campaign to develop and promote safer packaging for over-the-counter drugs. Dilenschneider (1990) summed up his power triangle by saying that you "must do worthy things, communicate sound messages, and seek recognition *quietly.*"

Public relations is that part of marketing involving promotion and publicity. Its components are the three legs of the power triangle—communication, recognition, and influence. PR may be needed in times of crisis to offset negative publicity, but it should also be an ongoing function, to promote positive action within the company and the community.

## ADVERTISING

Like public relations, advertising is also promotion. Usually we think of advertising as something a company pays for and PR as "free." This isn't necessarily the case. Examples of "free" advertising abound, and companies are certainly spending a good deal on PR campaigns. We will consider them separately, but the line between them is blurred.

Advertising is a fascinating and creative field, one lending itself easily to retrospective analysis. As consumers, we have all had opportunities to view the best and worst, the successes and flops, of brand advertising for consumer goods.

A few spectacular and well-publicized failures come easily to mind. For example, in the 1980s, when Coca-Cola dominated the soft drink market, the company introduced "New Coke." Although the product had done well in market tests, it was, in the end, a disaster. Coca-Cola lost a significant market share (that it has not completely regained) and some credibility among consumers (Oliver, 1986). Although the failure of this product cannot be blamed entirely on advertising, a different approach might have saved the brand.

Some successful ads have failed to sell products. AlkaSeltzer, for example, once used a series of ads that featured a cartoon stomach talking about its problems and the benefits of drinking AlkaSeltzer. These creative, award-winning ads were funny; people liked them. Unfortunately, the talking stomach everybody liked didn't sell the product and the campaign was abandoned.

Sometimes advertising works very well for products the public might be better off without. The Marlboro man cigarette ads are a classic example. Marlboro was one of the first cigarettes with a filter. When the brand was introduced, it was marketed as a mild cigarette for women and didn't sell well. When Marlboro switched over to the rugged, manly, outdoors theme, the brand took off and dominated the cigarette market for years, using the same ad theme for decades.

Advertising must be specific to the product or service's market segment. Fast food is an example of a product (and service) used by the general public, and like soft drink ads, fast-food advertising must reach a wide audience. McDonald's offers a good example of segment-specific advertising. Its goal is clearly to bring as many people as possible into its restaurants, and the company has successfully sold billions of hamburgers. McDonald's advertising, however, is not aimed at "every man." Instead, it uses many different advertising messages to appeal to many different market segments: children (during Saturday morning cartoon time), teenagers, seniors, African Americans, and young working adults, to name a few.

What do these examples tell us about advertising? That it is a tricky business. A successful ad campaign involves a lot more than just a clever concept—it involves careful and detailed research. Consumers are inconsistent. About the only thing that most advertisers agree on is that it is very difficult to predict consumer response. Advertising shouldn't stand alone, but must be part of the overall marketing strategy.

## Planning

Where should you begin with advertising? With a strategic plan and its component, the marketing plan. Some marketing plans will rely heavily on advertising and others will not. Marketing and advertising objectives and budget should be developed as part of the planning process. Although you may find examples of successful advertising that was developed almost spontaneously, the most effective use of your advertising dollars will be achieved by having a plan, which follows your strategic objectives, and sticking to it.

## Research

Planning advertising requires research. Much of that research may be part of the development of the overall marketing plan, such as identifying the market niche for the product or service. Advertising research can be used to determine which ad messages or media work best in a specific market. The effectiveness of a given ad or ad campaign will need to be evaluated. Information gathered in advance of or to assess the effectiveness of advertising should also be shared with other members of the marketing group. The advertising research may reinforce existing data or contradict it, but it can prove valuable in either case.

Many firms specialize in market research. Some companies do their own research, even if it is quite sophisticated. One widely used form of market research is the focus group. A focus group is a small group of 5–10 people who meet the exact profile of the target market. They are brought together and, with a facilitator, discuss various marketing aspects of the product or service. Their emotional input is solicited. The facilitator is briefed in advance and the meetings are usually recorded (audio and/or video). Focus groups have also been used to develop ideas for new products or to determine new ways to use existing products. In either case, the use of focus groups has generally proven to be successful. They are also relatively low cost, so that even small businesses can afford to use focus groups.

## Media

Advertising media may refer to print media, such as newspapers or magazines. Print media also includes special interest magazines (the trade press), telephone yellow pages, newsletters, billboards, and other forms that deliver a message in writing, with or without pictures. Broadcast media includes radio and television—both of which are no longer just "mass media." Cable TV has brought about the development of highly specialized networks or stations, appealing to specific audiences. For example, most cable subscribers have access to a local information channel that may feature items of interest only to one county, and some cable networks specialize in music only, comedy only, even medicine only. Radio markets have become almost equally specialized, some going to talk-only formats, for example.

Media time or space can be purchased in different ways. Space in print media is usually sold by size, for example, by numbers of lines, column inches, or page or portion of a page. Media time is purchased in minutes, or fractions or multiples of minutes. Most media purchases include discounts for quantity, based on size (of print ads) or length (of TV ads) or on frequency (the numbers of ads purchased over a period of time) or some combination. You may negotiate with the seller directly, go through a purchasing service, or have your advertising agency buy space or time for you. A purchasing service or agency is usually paid indirectly, by purchasing the space or time at a discount and then reselling it to advertisers at full price.

The art of successful advertising includes choosing the right place to advertise, after you have chosen the best media. For example, in print media you have a choice of many different magazines catering to the same market. Within each publication, you have a choice of where in the magazine to put the ad (front, back, pull-out, opposite editorial content, etc.), and if your ad is less than a full page, you can specify where on the page it appears. Good placement begins during the planning process but also involves research. Even the best planning and research isn't perfect and you may to have use trial and error. This can be costly, however, so planning and research are important.

## Direct Mail

Another form of advertising, with which everyone with a mailbox is familiar, is direct mail. Catalogs are one form of sales by direct mail and can be thought of as large ads. Although many people find "junk mail" a nuisance at one time or another, it is a highly successful marketing tool. Easy access to computer technology has made sophisticated databases for mailing list management available to a wide range of users, from huge companies to one-person operations.

One major advantage of direct mail is that it offers the advertiser a method for delivering a message to a highly focused group. Direct mail can be more cost effective than mass media. Even if you are trying to reach a mass market, your advertising may be more successful if you divide the market into specific segments and tailor a message to each segment. With direct mail, you can be sure that you are only paying to send your message to qualified individuals. Making sure they see the message has become the challenge.

Evaluating the effectiveness of advertising can be difficult. If the goal of advertising is to create sales, then a good way to evaluate the effectiveness of an ad is to track the sales it generates. Sometimes this is nearly impossible, but using direct mail simplifies the task of tracking the source of each sale.

## Displays

Point-of-purchase displays and trade shows are other commonly used advertising methods. These techniques are closely related to both advertising and sales. Point-of-purchase displays are frequently used to promote consumer products. Appearing at the end of aisles or checkout counters in retail stores, these displays are successful for products where brand decisions are most often made in the store. These displays are also used to deliver health promotion messages, as evidenced by the displays of brochures in the reception areas or treatment rooms of many healthcare practices. Point-of-purchase displays may also include samples or tie in with posters.

Trade shows are exhibits open to members of a specific trade, profession, or interest group. One of their main advantages is that, like direct mail, they reach a very specific audience. Some trade shows (usually for an entire industry) allow selling and others do not. Companies participate in trade shows that prohibit direct selling for advertising or public relations purposes.

As you can tell from the examples used, advertising can encompass a wide range of activities. Each can be a specialization of its own, although one common denominator among successful advertising is specificity. Advertising messages have a better chance of success if they are aimed at a very specific segment of the market, sometimes referred to as a subsegment or market niche. To prepare this sort of message, you need to have a good understanding of the market niche and how your product or service fits the needs of that group. Although market research and ad development may best be left to the professionals, it is often the employees who have the most contact with customers who can provide some real insight into this relationship.

## Advertising and Healthcare Delivery

Very few people come into the field of healthcare delivery with a background in advertising. For this reason, probably very few healthcare providers are qualified to design advertising messages for healthcare markets. On the other hand, probably very few advertising professionals began their careers as healthcare providers, and so they may not understand the dynamics of the marketplace of healthcare delivery as well as someone who has been working with patients. In the end, success may require a careful collaboration between these experts to create an effective message.

Advertising can play an important role in healthcare—not in selling services, but in promoting health and selling the benefits of prevention. Although advertising professional services was once taboo, it is increasingly accepted. Whatever your views on this controversial issue, don't overlook the benefits of advertising the value of healthcare services and of promoting preventive behaviors.

# SALES

Selling is persuading the customer to buy your product or to use your service. Sales can be considered from different perspectives. Some sales are direct from the company and others are indirect, involving third parties. You may be selling products, services, or some combination of the two.

Sales, advertising, and public relations are all closely related. For example, some makers of athletic shoes use professional athletes to endorse their products. Having the athletes wear the shoes during games is public relations—no direct sales pitch is being made, but communication is taking place. The brand of shoe is being positioned in the public eye as being associated with winning at athletics. Some of these athletes also appear in commercials promoting the shoes. This is advertising. Although the athletes do not make sales calls at shoe stores, their professional endorsements have generally been effective in increasing sales.

## Direct Sales

Every business has a customer or client, even if that client is internal. At some point, a product or service is delivered to someone. Selling may be handled directly by the company in a variety of ways, by mail, by phone, by sales call, or by some combination of these methods.

### MAIL

As already mentioned, sales may be made by direct mail. In this case, your mailing may be your advertising as well as your sales tool. Some direct mail companies also use their mailings to recruit new customers. Have you ever received a catalog with an offer to "send one to a friend"? In this case, the mail piece was used for advertising, selling, and PR. A key point with direct mail selling is making the purchase easy for the customer because there won't be any salesperson present to help with the purchase. For example, almost all catalogs take all major credit cards and have toll-free lines for ordering.

### TELEPHONE

Telemarketing is big business. It combines many of the advantages of direct mail, such as highly targeted audiences, with the speed and efficiency of the telephone, and it offers direct, personal contact. Of course, not all products or services lend themselves to this type of approach and many customers do not like it. Telemarketing is also used in areas other than sales, for example, in conducting market research or in public relations.

### IN-HOUSE SALES FORCE

An in-house sales force is composed of salespeople who are employed by your company, as opposed to manufacturers' representatives or distributors (discussed in the next section). The sales force may require a considerable amount of support and, in exchange, can be of great value to the company. The sales force will require some type of management and other personnel support, depending on its size, as well as office space, equipment, and presentation or sales materials. The sales staff may install or service point-of-purchase displays and also be involved with trade shows or meetings. Salespeople can be a valuable source of market information, although it may be biased. By the nature of the job, salespeople are in constant contact with customers. Such communication can be used not just for sales, but for informal market research and for public relations as well.

## Indirect Sales

Depending on the field, a business may not use an in-house sales force or sell directly to the public, but may instead rely on indirect sales methods, such as manufacturers' representatives, distributors, retailers, or some combination of methods, direct or indirect.

### MANUFACTURERS' REPRESENTATIVES

Manufacturers' representatives (reps) are usually independent sales organizations. They may represent only one client or, more often, they sell the products of different manufacturers in a similar industry to a group of similar clients. They are usually paid a commission on the sales made in the territory which by agreement is theirs. The particulars may vary from company to company.

### DISTRIBUTORS

Distributors are most often associated with retail (direct sales to the public) businesses, such as grocery and clothing stores. Distributors are often referred to as the "middlemen." They buy products from producers, or other distributors, and resell them to retail stores. They buy at a discount and sell at a higher rate. Their profit margin (see Chapter 3) is the difference. As with other types of sales arrangements, there are many variations on this scheme, depending on the needs of the businesses involved.

### RETAIL

Whether you love shopping or hate it, everyone is familiar with retail. These are the businesses that sell directly to the public. Usually retail operations are located in stores, although there are plenty of examples of businesses that sell direct without having stores, such as mail order catalogs. Like distributors, they buy in volume, at a discount, and sell at a higher rate. Their profit margin is the difference. For some retail businesses, jewelry for example, the profit margin may be as high as 300%. For others, it is very low. Grocery stores, for instance, sometimes operate at margins below 1%.

### PRODUCTS, SERVICES, AND CUSTOMERS

Products or services are what businesses sell. Most businesses provide neither one exclusively. Management expert Tom Peters (1987) and others have focused management thinking on the connection between products and services. Customers are buying solutions to problems. This often means that companies that are selling products must also offer service and support to go with the products in order to deliver the value that customers are seeking. Some companies that are primarily in the service sector have also been seeking ways to offer products so that customers may find a more complete solution to their problems available from one source. This type of diversification requires a careful balancing act. While it is important to offer your customers a complete solution, no business can be all things to all people. It is better to do a few things extraordinarily well than to do many things in a haphazard fashion.

Satisfied customers are a must. Without them no business can survive for long. Most businesses want to make repeat sales to customers, to make marketing efforts more cost effective. Furthermore, making only one sale per customer can be a hard way to do business, whereas satisfied repeat customers should be easier to sell to than new customers. In a service business, repeat sales are vital. You want the client to return to use your service more than once and to refer others. A business also needs satisfied customers so that products that have been sold are not returned.

Long-term successful selling involves service and support. Some terms that reflect this sales and service attitude are customer-driven marketing and total customer satisfaction. If the entire organization is oriented toward being market driven and responsive to customers, everyone is in sales, even if they do not have direct contact with clients. Production, quality control, accounting, and all functions or departments impact the quality or timeliness of delivery of products or services. Sales are the front line.

Sales is often approached from the standpoint of what the company is selling. A better focus for sales, and marketing in general, is "what is the customer buying?" Customers may be buying your product to get the service that comes with it and as such regard their purchases as solutions to problems rather than as items or professional advice. The function of marketing is getting the right product to the right customers at the right price at the right time. Such a function involves identifying the customer and the market and defining the three P's for the product or service.

## Summary

Marketing creates markets, customers, and products. Public relations makes potential customers aware of your company and its members, products, or services. Advertising creates a demand for your products or services. Selling gets the consumer to purchase or use your particular service or product. Marketing is the business function that coordinates all these activities.

## Review Questions

1. Define marketing.

2. Define the three P's of marketing.

3. Give an example of a product you are familiar with which has positioned itself in different market segments by changing its position, price, or promotion. Explain how the change was accomplished.

4. Define public relations.

5. Give an example of a public relations campaign and explain why it was a success or failure.

6. Define advertising.

7. Give an example of how advertising might have a positive effect on a business or project with which you are involved.

8. Define sales.

9. Using a business or project with which you are involved as an example, explain whether or not customers' needs are being met and how. If the current methods are not successful, how might they be changed?

10. Describe the purpose of marketing management.

## SUGGESTED READING

Hiam, A., & Schewe, C. D. (1992). *The portable MBA in marketing.* New York: John Wiley & Sons.

Mayer, M. (1991). *Whatever happened to Madison Avenue? Advertising in the '90s.* Boston: Little, Brown.

Nichols, J. E. (1990). *By the numbers: Using demographics and psychographics for business growth in the, '90s.* Chicago: Bonus Books.

## REFERENCES

Davis, R. (1990). Marketing management: Becoming a market-driven company. In *The portable MBA,* edited by E. Collins and M. A. Devanna, pp. 174–218. New York: John Wiley & Sons.

Dilenschneider, R. (1990). *Power and influence: Mastering the art of persuasion.* New York: Prentice-Hall, pp. 5, 159–170.

Ogilvy, D. (1983). *Ogilvy on advertising.* New York: Crown Publishers. p. 172.

Oliver, T. (1986). *The Real Coke, the Real Story.* New York: Random House.

Peters, T. (1987). *Thriving on chaos.* New York: Alfred A. Knopf.

# CHAPTER 5

# Quality

---

## *Objectives*

After reading this chapter and completing the review questions, the reader should be able to:

- Define quality control, quality assurance, quality circles, and total quality management.
- Discuss the client's role in total quality management of oral healthcare delivery.
- Give three examples of total quality management of oral healthcare delivery in action.
- Define the three types of quality assurance standards.
- Describe an evaluation mechanism for three types of quality assurance standards.
- Describe how a code of ethics might be used in business.
- Discuss an example of a manager's role in resolving an ethical dilemma.

---

Although this chapter is the last one in this section, quality should be the first priority. It was necessary to present the information in Chapters 1–4 first to provide background for the discussion of quality. Managing for quality cannot be overlooked or taken for granted and must be an integral part of all management functions. Quality cannot come from management alone, however. Every staff member must share a common understanding of the practice's mission and commitment to quality.

Quality is the key in all areas of management. Managing for production is not enough. The quality of services or goods produced is at least as important as the quantity.

## TERMS

Some of the current terms used in managing for quality include quality control (QC), quality assurance (QA), quality circles, continuous quality improvement (CQI), and total quality management (TQM). One definition of total quality management is "making customer satisfaction the number one priority" (Port and Smith 1992). Systems that emphasize quality standards based on customer perception have given rise to such terms as total customer responsiveness, customer orientation, and customer-driven organization. More are being introduced all the time.

*Quality control* is a term often used in industry to describe methods of checking and inspecting products as they are assembled to detect any errors. The process may also include testing the final product to be sure that it operates according to standard specifications. Quality control procedures usually involve defining specific standards and tolerance limits that partial assemblies or completed products must meet to be acceptable for release. Quality control can be achieved in a variety of ways. For example, some businesses have committees of employees, managers, or a combination of the two to review safety or product defects. A review board may monitor quality, customer satisfaction, or competence. Some health organizations have patient advocates to assist the quality assurance committee.

*Quality assurance* is a term more often associated with the service sector, for which it is often difficult to define specific standards. In healthcare, the standard of care is frequently defined as the usual and customary acceptable treatment. Standards of care are usually applied to a community or local area, so that the standard of care in New York City may not be the same as the standard in Rome, Georgia. Professional groups may develop standards of care to serve as quality assurance guidelines. Hospitals and other large institutions may have their own quality assurance standards, in addition to the usual and customary or those of any professional group. In this case, a specific group within the institution may be assigned to assure compliance with the standards.

*Quality circles* are sometimes used to implement quality assurance/quality control (QA/QC) programs. As the name implies, the purpose of quality circles is to include all aspects of service, production, and management in the QA/QC program in an equal and *ongoing* basis. As illustrated in Figure 5.1, the quality circle includes QA/QC as part of the process or cycle, rather than as something separate and apart from it.

The rationale for including QA/QC as part of all production or service operations is so that quality is evaluated continually, rather than at the end of the process or just occasionally. In this way, everyone involved is working to achieve a consistent standard of quality. If errors are made or standards are not met, these problems will be identified and corrected sooner and, hopefully, by the very people responsible for making the error. If QA/QC occurs apart from the service or production arena, quality is being judged by some outside party and errors are discovered much later in the process, when they may be more difficult or impossible to correct.

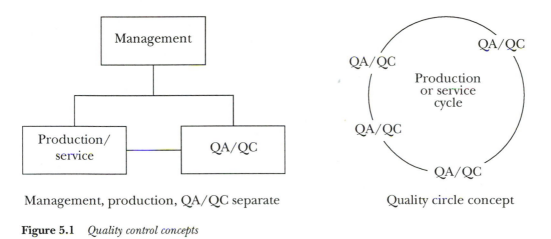

Management, production, QA/QC separate        Quality circle concept

**Figure 5.1** *Quality control concepts*

When QA/QC is separated from service or production, those responsible for doing the work may feel resentment at being judged by those in QA/QC. This is not conducive to improvement. When workers are responsible for evaluating their own output, they are more likely to accept responsibility for errors and to be more willing to improve.

*Continuous quality improvement* is a related concept. As the name implies, the purpose of CQI is to integrate QA/QC into all operations, so that quality is being improved continuously. To implement a system of CQI, you must have specific quality standards and the total organization must be involved in the ongoing process consistently.

Briefly, the objectives of *total quality management* are reduced cycle time and defect elimination. Cycle time runs from the beginning of a service or process, such as bringing a product to market, to the end, and defect elimination means those products or services are delivered error free. TQM systems aim to reduce cycle time and eliminate defects by applying all available measures, but especially through employee empowerment and CQI. An important point of TQM is that reduced cycle time and defect elimination go together. It is not the aim of TQM to achieve one without the other. These goals are ambitious, yet multitudes of organizations, large and small, have successfully implemented TQM programs. Implementing TQM involves the entire corporate culture (attitudes, beliefs, people, and other resources). These systems may start with top management, but they cannot succeed unless all the organization's leaders (both official and unofficial) and members are completely a part of the process. Remember, the goal is *total* quality.

Total quality management and related terms, such as total customer responsiveness, emphasize quality standards based on client satisfaction. The focus is external, rather than internal. Businesses, for-profit or not-for-profit, exist to serve their clients, by delivering either services or products or both. It is logical therefore that the clients should define the level of quality they expect. This does not mean that businesses go out and ask their clients to write quality standards. It does mean that *everyone* in the organization listens to its clients carefully and makes infinite adjustments to assure that clients are completely satisfied.

# QUALITY AND HEALTHCARE DELIVERY

What does total quality management mean for oral healthcare delivery? Healthcare consumers must set the standards for their care. Practitioners must provide treatment that is technically correct, explain treatment options and prognoses to clients, and let clients make informed decisions about their own care. Managers and clinicians must listen and understand what their clients' priorities are. Priorities will differ from market to market. Probably very few clients will come to the dental hygienist asking for perfectly smooth root surfaces free of all toxins, but they may ask for shorter or longer appointments, or evening or Saturday appointments. They may ask for brighter smiles or fresh breath. They may be seeking oral healthcare that is integrated with their total health. Listen to what clients ask for and provide that.

A focus on client-oriented standards is a new concept for healthcare providers. In the past, professionals decided what the standard of care should be, based on their own expertise. They assumed that patients, with no training in the complexities of healthcare, did not know what was best for them. In dental hygiene, this internal focus resulted in standards that emphasized providing technically perfect services (e.g., flawlessly smooth root surfaces) even though most clients could hardly tell the difference between a perfect root and an imperfect one. Most clients do not choose an oral healthcare provider based on a knowledgeable assessment of the provider's technical ability. Clients base their quality evaluations on their own value systems.

Clients who present with periodontal disease and ask for fresh breath may need root planing and antimicrobial treatment to achieve that treatment goal (fresh breath). This treatment may also satisfy the hygienist's goal (periodontal health). Those clients will value a treatment outcome of periodontal health only if they understand how root planing and fresh breath are related. Clients who present with periodontal disease and ask for whiter teeth may never value periodontal therapy unless uncontrolled disease leads to noticeable cosmetic changes and tooth loss. Even in this situation, dentures, regardless of functional limitations, may be more esthetically pleasing to the clients than the natural teeth will ever be. It is the client's right to make an *informed* choice.

Making an informed choice does not mean blindly doing what the client asks. For example, if a client, when informed of her periodontal status, says, "I want dentures," the clinician does not hand her the oral surgeon's card and say, "Make an appointment with the dentist next week." The client needs to be informed regarding the dental diagnosis, treatment options, and the approximate costs and limitations of various treatments options. This discussion need not be lengthy *if* the client has a few questions. The client does have a right to have all her questions answered before making a choice. Even the client with many questions doesn't need an information dump. She needs answers she can understand.

Consider a scenario where a client makes a choice not in keeping with the values of her dentist. A 60-year-old woman, in good health, makes an emergency visit to her dentist because of an abscessed molar. The dentist evaluates the tooth and concludes that the client's oral health is generally good and that the molar can be saved by performing a root canal. The dentist explains the disadvantages of losing the molar and all the client's treatment options. The client wants the tooth extracted. She believes that she will lose all her teeth eventually, just as her friends and family have, and doesn't see any point in spending hundreds of dollars delaying the inevitable. The client informs the dentist that she will go home and think about it. What the client thinks is that the dentist is trying to sell her something she doesn't need or want. Her evaluation of the quality of this dentist's services will be that the dentist is only in it for the money, when the dentist has only tried to provide the client with the best possible care.

There is no right or wrong to either of these views. This dentist may not be able to accept this client's value judgment. If this is the case, the dentist is probably better off losing this client. Providing for her, and others with similar values, the treatment she requests will create internal conflict and dissatisfaction for this dentist. This stress will affect other areas of the dentist's practice and life. If, however, the dentist wants to serve this segment of the market, she will have to accept that this client and her peers do not see preventive treatment the same way she does, but are nonetheless entitled to make decisions about their own healthcare. This is total customer responsiveness.

Total quality management should also be the basis for your marketing. You must know who your clients are and meet their needs to the letter. Most practices will serve a number of micro markets. If your office is computerized, your on-line client records will contain most of the demographic information you need for defining your micro markets. Part of the planning process will involve choosing which markets to pursue and which to drop. If a practice is to be competitive, it cannot be all things to all people. A few clients may not meet any of your market profiles, but stay with the practice anyway. (These clients can point the way to new market niches.)

Let your clients decide what services you will provide and how. Finding a need and filling it is much easier than deciding whom you want to serve and then attracting them. Value judgments are involved in making these choices, however. If your values conflict with most of your clients', and those clients are setting the standards for your practice, you will never be satisfied in your job. You cannot easily change the values of your clients, but you may be able to find new market segments to serve or you may need to find a new job.

How can you be totally responsive to your clients? Many attributes attract clients to particular practices. Some of these common features are discussed here for illustration, not in any particular order. Which will be most important to your practice? Ask your clients. Their quality issues may not even be mentioned here. Find out what *your* clients want and give it to them.

Unless you are choosing a location for a new practice or new job, location may not be something you have a lot of choice about. It may, however, influence the market segments available to the practice. For example, a practice located in the midst of a city business district or suburban industrial zone will have mostly working adults as clients. If many of the clients are white-collar office workers, they will want appointments early in the morning and during the evening and weekends. If many of your clients come from a nearby factory that runs on shifts, you may have peak hours of demand at the start and end of each shift.

If you are in a general practice located in a semirural area surrounded by many large families, you will have clients of all ages. This may seem ideal (many markets) at first glance, but the total population is limited because of the rural location. You may have to identify the largest two or three micro markets and appeal to these segments by accommodating their requirements.

Convenient hours are a frequent request. Convenience will depend on the particulars of your micro markets. In the preceding example, where several micro markets were adult professionals, the practice required evening and weekend hours. It can be difficult to attract the best people to work these hours unless you are responsive to employee needs. Some people will gladly work evenings and weekends for higher pay or extra benefits. The secret is to find a negotiating point. If your clients need evening hours, you can find a way to satisfy them. Paying employees more for evenings, weekends, or holidays may mean that the you have to charge higher fees, either at these times, or in general, depending on what the market can bear. If no one else in your area is offering evening hours, you can get away with charging more for evenings. If a number of practices around you offer evening hours, however, your clients may not be willing to pay special evening rates at your practice. Ask them!

No one is going to volunteer to pay higher fees for no good reason. However, if clients find a service that they need (i.e., evening hours), they will value it enough to pay a little extra. Those who can't afford or don't need to pay extra for the evening appointments may be able to make time to come in during the off-peak hours and save money. This might appeal to families. No one in the practice, though, can take a guess at what clients want and are willing to pay for. You must listen to what they ask for and provide that. You do not need marketing ideas from books or magazines. You need marketing ideas from your clients and information from many sources (especially employees) on how to implement them.

Your facility is another marketing point. If you are located in a plush office building in downtown Manhattan and decorate your office with industrial grade carpet and crate-style furniture, you are probably sending a negative message to your upscale clients. They are used to having luxury accommodations and paying for them. If your practice has an institutional or clinic feel, it may reflect on the quality of your services in their eyes. On the other hand, if your practice is in a rural, farm community and you have Chippendale chairs, Persian rugs, and original oil paintings in your reception area, your patients may begin to wonder if your fees are too high. Again, this depends on the clients. If you are in horse farm country in Middleburg, Virginia, and are trying to appeal to the well-to-do horse crowd, this decor might work well.

The personalities of all employees need to match your clients' needs. It is certainly possible, and desirable, for many different types of people to coexist harmoniously. The entire staff need not be like the clients, but only to treat them respectfully and make them feel valued. If you are in a rural practice, everyone does not have to pretend to be a country bumpkin to get along with clients, but the staff member who treats clients condescendingly will cause problems—loss of clients and loss of referrals. An employee in an upscale urban practice who thinks most of the clients are supercilious snobs will alienate them quickly and the practice will suffer accordingly.

Some clients will be concerned about skills and technology. With so much media attention focused on infection control, most clients will probably be reassured to know that everyone on staff is up to date on infection-control procedures. Let them know that all of you are involved in continuing education, are aware of the latest standards, and are following them. The practice owners should not be whining to clients about the costs of compliance or listing reasons why the practice doesn't need to comply. Clients are not concerned with your profit margins but about safe, effective healthcare. While it might be politically expedient to explain what is wrong with infection control policy, discussing this with clients may leave them wondering which standards the practice is complying with and which it is ignoring and just how this is affecting the safety of their treatment. Your practice should be meeting your clients' needs. Most clients want treatment in a safe environment that meets the highest government standards, whatever they are, even if this means that every staff member wears a pink hair net and puts on a fresh one in front of every client.

In some markets, clients want state-of-the-art treatment and in others clients fear fads. Almost without exception, you must let your clients know about ongoing staff development, training, and continuing education. Show them with your actions, positive comments, attention to detail, and interest in their needs and feedback. This will emphasize your overall commitment to quality, but does not mean that you must emphasize that you are using new procedures if your clients don't value new technology. Clients are paying for your professional expertise and expect you to be up to date in your training. They may or may not want to try the latest materials, mouth rinses, or laser treatments. You should be aware of current developments in your field, but you may not want to market them aggressively. Supply what your clients ask for. If 10 people come in one week asking about antimicrobial periodontal therapy, this should identify a trend. Your micro market may be changing or you may have attracted a new group. If you don't have all the technical information you need, get it quickly. If clients are asking for this therapy, have it available.

You may not need a highly structured system for documenting client requests. Just keep a list in areas where you interact with clients and compile those lists weekly. Have one person or group review them regularly and use the information to guide your planning.

The quality of the communications your practice has with clients may be what they remember most readily. Communications include how everyone talks to and treats clients while they are in your office or on the phone. You are also communicating nonverbally with clients when they visit. If your reception area is cold, sterile, cramped, impersonal, walled off by glass from the rest of the office, what message are you sending? Your decor and your equipment tell the client volumes about the practice. If you are a family-oriented practice and you have no chairs or toys for children, are you really asking children to come to your practice? Would children be more interested in visiting a practice with video games or with *Time* magazines in the reception area? If seniors or retired people form part of your important markets, they may not appreciate rap music and video games. You may be able to provide areas or appointment times appropriate for many different micro markets with a little planning.

Print communications deserve careful attention because these often reach clients at home and may stay around for some time. Printed items include bills, statements, letters, newsletters, personal notes, appointment reminders, advertising, business cards, anything in print associated with your practice. Remember that your printed communications don't need to meet your standards of taste, but to meet your clients' standards. You will not be using these materials to wallpaper your home but to communicate to your clients just how valuable they are to you. You may need several different versions of the same piece to use with different micro markets. You may need to research and test to find the most effective, appealing message and style.

Have you ever wondered why some practitioners become involved in cosmetic procedures in a big way and always seem to be talking about how great it is? Making a large-scale change in a practice can be intimidating to the staff, requires additional training and equipment, and can involve exacting and time-consuming procedures. Yet these practices have some of the most highly motivated employees and great revenues. The big motivator for staff, and the big draw for clients, is that these practices are giving clients what they want—bright, photogenic smiles and improved self-image. Because cosmetic services frequently are not covered by insurance, some clients are spending a fortune out of pocket but are happy to go to the dentist. Client satisfaction motivates employees—they are not just slaving away for pennies on their paychecks. Their clients love them and are happy about the treatment they receive. Is there magic in cosmetic dentistry? No. There's magic in giving people what they want, in identifying needs and filling them. While we all need to meet the quality assurance standards of our professions, these must be only the foundation for meeting the quality standards of our clients.

# QUALITY ASSURANCE MECHANISMS

Quality assurance is a hot topic in medicine and nursing. Although it is certainly discussed in dentistry and dental hygiene, quality assurance and quality assurance mechanisms have not been discussed to the same extent as they have been in medicine and nursing. For example, the *Comprehensive Index to Nursing and Allied Health* (*CINAL*) is an index to all the journal articles printed in publications related to nursing and allied health. The *Index to Dental Literature* (*IDL*) is a similar index listing for dental and dental hygiene literature. Comparing the past three years of both these indexes reveals that CINAL lists an average of about 200 references under the heading Quality Assurance. Conversely, the IDL has an average of about 20 quality assurance references. This is an indicator of the difference between these fields with regard to their emphasis on quality assurance. There may be many reasons for this difference, but the result is that quality assurance standards are less well defined in oral healthcare.

Standards are one of the most controversial subjects in quality assurance. In evaluating quality, the establishment of the objective standards you need for comparison is always a sticking point. Some group or individual must define the standard of care that all practitioners must meet and it is difficult to get numbers of individuals to agree on a set of standards, let alone to get groups to agree. This is one of the points that is especially difficult in oral healthcare because the majority of practitioners are in solo or small practices, as compared to medicine and nursing where practitioners work more frequently in large groups, such as hospitals. The professions working more often in large groups are forced to come to some mutual understanding in order to proceed with business. The preponderance of literature on the subject in CINAL would at least indicate that nurses discuss the subject more often. Furthermore, the federal government is more closely involved with QA in medicine because of its financial interest in Medicare and Medicaid programs. This also fuels the drive toward more consistent evaluation standards and methods. Some private, managed dental care plans, PPOs, and HMOs have quality assurance programs, and provider participation is often mandatory.

Quality assurance standards can be created for several different aspects of healthcare delivery. Most commonly, these are divided into structure, process, and outcomes. Structural standards cover the setting, facility, equipment, human resources, and organization. Process standards cover the techniques and actions of actual delivery of care. Outcome standards cover the effects of treatment on client health and quality of life. Each of these areas contributes to the total healthcare delivery environment and each must be considered in developing a set of comprehensive quality assurance standards.

Establishing the standards may be the easiest part of the job. More difficult than writing standards is developing evaluation mechanisms. Evaluation mechanisms are necessary to determine whether established QA standards are being met. Some mechanisms of QA evaluation include site visits, chart audits, peer review, and networking. There are limitations to applying any of these to private dental practices.

Site visits can be useful for evaluating a practice's ability to meet structural standards and are used most often for hospitals and large HMOs. The facility being evaluated performs a self-evaluation and then a team of calibrated inspectors visits the facility and collects data for evaluation. This information can also be used by the facility as a basis for upgrading weak areas. Formal organizations involved in QA evaluation activities, such as the Joint Commission on Accreditation of Healthcare Organizations (JCAHO), may act as accrediting bodies for facilities. More than one evaluation method will be used.

Chart audits involve groups of calibrated examiners reviewing client records (usually a random sample) and recording the information. These audits are most useful for evaluating process of care, and long-range outcomes, especially those related to quality of life, may not be reflected in the client record. Chart audits are only as comprehensive and reliable as the information in the client records, which can often be limited, vague, and inconsistent.

Peer review can also be used to evaluate process of care and, to a limited extent, outcomes. Formal peer review is usually initiated by a complaint (from a provider, client, or insurance company) and then becomes a mediation process to settle the dispute. Networking, or study clubs, can be informal systems of peer review. As the name implies, peer review involves groups of like professionals evaluating one another. In a formal setting, a peer review committee or group may be formed for just this purpose. More informally, practitioners may visit one another's offices or exchange case studies. To accomplish any sort of peer review, you must have standards of comparison. The issues most often referred to peer review are process related, but structure and outcomes should also be considered, since all three of these are closely related. Information for evaluating outcomes may be found in client records. However, to gather data on long-range outcomes, some follow-up with clients is necessary and may involve examination of patients, interviews, or surveys.

There are limitations to each of these methods, though all have been used at some time in medicine. Methods other than peer review and networking involve the establishment of calibrated groups of reviewers. The training can be costly and time consuming, and most of these methods are time consuming for the organization being reviewed. All this adds to the total expensive of quality assurance programs. If you include the costs not only of work hours, but also of travel, equipment, and interruption of services during the review, the process can be prohibitively expensive.

Oral healthcare may offer additional challenges in QA. A.L. Morris et al. (1989) refer to the American Dental Association's definition of quality assurance as "the assessment or measurement of, or judgment about, the quality of care and the implementation of any necessary changes to either maintain or improve the quality of care" in the introduction to their report on the impact of a quality assessment program on the practice behavior of general practitioners. Based on their landmark research, they conclude that "combining office assessment with a proactive quality assurance program can influence practitioners' behavior to produce patient care programs of higher quality." Maryniuk (1989) pointed out that "until quality assurance and quality assessment are linked to activities such as reimbursement, reduction in malpractice premiums, or relicensing, it may be very difficult to make any inroads" in moving toward implementation of quality assurance programs in oral healthcare.

## SUGGESTIONS FOR ACTION

Admittedly, there is currently no nationally accepted standard of oral healthcare or of dental hygiene care. This does not strip the dental hygiene profit center manager or dental practice manager of all power to establish quality standards within their organization nor does it remove the manager's responsibility to do so. Providing quality care should be an integral part of the strategic plan. As each piece of the plan is developed, from mission to goals, objectives, action plans, and performance evaluation objectives, quality should be a focal point.

The American Dental Hygienists' Association (ADHA 1993) has published a literature review, *Quality Assurance and Its Applications to the Delivery of Services Provided by Dental Hygienists*, that is an excellent reference and source of information pertinent to dental practice as well as dental hygiene practice. It covers the ADHA *Standards of Applied Dental Hygiene Practice* (developed in 1986) and other models of healthcare quality assurance, standards of practice, and continuous quality improvement.

Although there are no "official" standards, you can create your own performance standards and they need not apply to any other practice. It is important to have measurable standards in place to keep everyone focused on quality. As the old saying goes, "What gets measured gets done." In an evaluation of the impact of a quality assessment program developed by the ADA, long-term follow-up of the 300 volunteer practices showed that those participating in the program demonstrated a significant increase in quality (Morris et al. 1989). Just having the QA program in place had a positive impact on the practitioners' behavior.

Your in-office QA standards should measure observable actions, behaviors, or outcomes. Writing QA standards is like writing performance objectives. To use the standards for evaluation, you must be able to observe whether the standards are being met, using criteria based on your strategic plan and, most importantly, on client perception. As discussed earlier, the most important measure of quality you can have is client satisfaction. Internally, you may need standards of technical performance as well, but the highest priority should be given to treatment outcomes satisfying to patients and improving the quality of their lives (as measured by their standards, not yours).

Infection control is one area in which you must have QA standards equal to or higher than those of the government (OSHA, etc.). Most clients will not have the expertise necessary to define infection control standards, but most will probably be satisfied if your practice meets or exceeds government standards. If there is a lot of public concern about infection control, listen to your clients to discover what they need to see, hear, and know about infection control to allay all their fears.

Comprehensive care is a quality issue. Everyone in your practice must work to ensure that all clients are given the opportunity to discuss and understand their comprehensive healthcare needs. It will be beyond the scope of any practice to treat all their healthcare needs, and some clients may choose to ignore some of their healthcare needs. You should, however, have standards that establish your services as an integral part of the clients' total healthcare.

# ETHICS

No discussion of business management would be complete without considering ethics. Managers face many ethical dilemmas in their work and may also be involved in resolving the ethical dilemmas of their employees and clients. Ethics is a complex field, affecting all areas of our lives. A complete discussion of this topic, even as it relates to oral healthcare delivery, is far beyond the scope of this text. The following discussion is limited to examples of codes of ethics and a discussion of management roles in resolving ethical dilemmas.

## Codes of Ethics

Most professional associations have codes of ethics. The codes of the American Dental Hygienists' Association (1992; currently under revision), and the American Dental Association (1991) follow. They may or may not cover the needs of your practice. If they do not seem to apply, you can establish your own code or ethical statement for use by everyone in your practice.

### PRINCIPLES OF ETHICS OF THE AMERICAN DENTAL HYGIENISTS' ASSOCIATION

Each member of the American Dental Hygienists' Association has the ethical obligation to subscribe to the following principles:

- To provide oral healthcare utilizing highest professional knowledge, judgment and ability.
- To serve all patients without discrimination.
- To hold professional patient relationships in confidence.
- To utilize every opportunity to increase public understanding of oral health practices.
- To generate public confidence in members of the dental health profession.
- To cooperate with all health professions in meeting the health needs of the public.
- To recognize and uphold the laws and regulations governing this profession.
- To participate responsibly in this professional Association and uphold its purpose.
- To maintain professional competence through continuing education.
- To exchange professional knowledge with other health professions.
- To represent dental hygiene with high standards of personal conduct.
  [ADHA, 1992]

## AMERICAN DENTAL ASSOCIATION, PRINCIPLES OF ETHICS AND CODE OF PROFESSIONAL CONDUCT

1. Service to the Public and Quality of Care
   The dentist's primary professional obligation shall be service to the public. The competent and timely delivery of quality care within the bounds of the clinical circumstance presented by the patient, with due consideration being given to the needs and desires of the patient, shall be the most important aspect of that obligation.
   1.A.  Patient Selection
   While dentists, in serving the public, may exercise reasonable discretion in selecting patients for their practices, dentists shall not refuse to accept patients into their practice or deny dental service to patients because of the patient's race, creed, color, sex, or national origin.
   1.B.  Patient Records
   Dentists are obliged to safeguard the confidentiality of patient records. Dentists shall maintain patient records in a manner consistent with the protection of the welfare of the patient. Upon request of a patient or another dental practitioner, dentists shall provide any information that will be beneficial for the future treatment of that patient.
   1.C.  Community Service
   Since dentists have an obligation to use their skills, knowledge, and experience for the improvement of the dental health of the public and are encouraged to be leaders in their community, dentists in such service shall conduct themselves in such a manner as to maintain or elevate the esteem of the profession.
   1.D.  Emergency Service
   Dentists shall be obliged to make reasonable arrangements for the emergency care of their patients of record. Dentists shall be obliged

when consulted in an emergency by patients not of record to make reasonable arrangements for emergency care. If treatment is provided, the dentist, upon completion of such treatment, is obliged to return the patient to his or her dentist unless the patient expressly reveals a different preference.

1.E.  Consultation and Referral

Dentists shall be obliged to seek consultation, if possible, whenever the welfare of patients will be safeguarded or advanced by utilizing those who have special skills, knowledge, and experience. When patients visit or are referred to specialists or consulting dentists for consultation:

1. The specialists or consulting dentists upon completion of their care shall return the patient, unless the patient expressly reveals a different preference, to the referring dentist, or if none, to the dentist of record for future care.

2. The specialists shall be obliged when there is no referring dentist and upon a completion of their treatment to inform patients when there is a need for further dental care.

1.F.  Use of Auxiliary Personnel

Dentists shall be obliged to protect the health of their patient by only assigning to qualified auxiliaries those duties which can legally be delegated. Dentists shall be further obliged to prescribe and supervise the work of all auxiliary personnel working under their direction and control.

1.G.  Justifiable Criticism

Dentists shall be obliged to report to the appropriate reviewing agency as determined by the local component or constituent society instances of gross or continual faulty treatment by other dentists. Patients should be informed of their present oral health status without disparaging comment about prior services. Dentists issuing public statement with respect to the profession shall have a reasonable basis to believe that the comments made are true.

1.H.  Expert Testimony

Dentists may provide expert testimony when that testimony is essential to a just and fair disposition of a judicial or administrative action.

1.I.  Rebate and Split Fees

Dentists shall not accept or tender rebates or split fees.

1.J.  Representation of Care

Dentists shall not represent the care being rendered in a false or misleading manner.

1.K.  Representation of Fees

Dentists shall not represent the fees being charged for providing care in a false or misleading manner.

1.L.  Patient Involvement

The dentist should inform the patient of the proposed treatment, and any reasonable alternatives, in a manner that allows the patient to become involved in treatment decision.

2. Education

   The privilege of dentists to be accorded professional status rests primarily in the knowledge, skill, and experience with which they serve their patients and society. All dentists, therefore, have the obligation of keeping their knowledge and skill current.

3. Government of a Profession

   Every profession owes society the responsibility to regulate itself. Such regulation is achieved largely through the influence of the professional societies. All dentists, therefore, have the dual obligation of making themselves a part of a professional society and of observing its rules of ethics.

4. Research and Development

   Dentists have the obligation of making the results and benefits of their investigative efforts available to all when they are useful in safeguarding or promoting the health of the public.

   4.A.  Devices and Therapeutic Methods

   Except for formal investigative studies, dentists shall be obliged to prescribe, dispense, or promote only those devices, drugs, and other agents whose complete formulae are available to the dental profession. Dentists shall have the further obligation of not holding out as exclusive any device, agent, methods, or technique.

   4.B.  Patents and Copyrights

   Patents and copyrights may be secured by dentists provided that such patents and copyrights shall not be used to restrict research or practice.

5. Professional Announcement

   In order to properly serve the public, dentists should represent themselves in a manner that contributes to the esteem of the profession. Dentists should not misrepresent their training and competence in any way that would be false or misleading in any respect.

   5.A.  Advertising

   Although any dentist may advertise, no dentist shall advertise or solicit patients in any form of communication in a manner that is false or misleading in any material respect.

   5.B.  Name of Practice

   Since the name under which a dentist conducts his or her practice may be a factor in the selection process of the patient, the use of a trade name or an assumed name that is false or misleading in any material respect is unethical. Use of the name of a dentist no longer actively associated with the practice may be continued for a period not to exceed one year.

   5.C.  Announcement of Specialization and Limitation of Practice

   This section and Section 5.D are designed to help the public make an informed selection between the practitioner who has completed an accredited program beyond the dental degree and a practitioner who has not completed such a program.

   The special areas of dental practice approved by the American Dental Association and the designation for ethical specialty announcement and limitation of practice are: dental public health, endodontics, oral pathology, oral and maxillofacial surgery, orthodontics, pediatric dentistry, periodontics, and prosthodontics.

Dentists who choose to announce specialization should use "specialist in" or "practice limited to" and shall limit their practice exclusively to the announced special area(s) of dental practice, provided at the time of the announcement such dentists have met in each approved specialty for which they announce the existing educational requirements and standards set forth by the American Dental Association.

Dentists who use their eligibility to announce as specialists to make the public believe that specialty services rendered in the dental office are being rendered by qualified specialists when such is not the case are engaged in unethical conduct. The burden of responsibility is on specialists to avoid any inference that general practitioners who are associated with specialists are qualified to announce themselves as specialists. [General standards and standards for multiple-specialty announcements are included.]

5.D.  General Practitioner Announcement of Services
General dentists who wish to announce the services available in their practices are permitted to announce the availability of those services so long as they avoid any communications that express or imply specialization. General dentists shall also state that the services are being provided by general dentists. No dentist shall announce available services in any way that would be false or misleading in any material respect. [ADA, 1991]

The ADA Code also includes extensive advisory opinions throughout that may serve as guidelines for interpretation of the code.

## Uses of Codes of Ethics

The purpose of establishing codes of ethics should not be to prescribe how to act in every possible situation, but rather to provide a framework for making ethical decisions. Useful codes give guidance on how to think, not what to think. Every businessperson will probably encounter some unimaginable situations in the course of a lifetime of work. The person who uses some ethical framework as a basis for action is, hopefully, more likely to make an ethical decision. It may not be necessary to have a written code, but they can be helpful. In a work situation, people from many different backgrounds are brought together and asked to function as a team in the same environment. Values and beliefs are based on life experience, so each of these people may bring a unique ethical perspective to your business. Everyone is entitled to their personal values and beliefs. A strong, quality-oriented organization needs people who share a common ethical code regarding business matters, and successful managers need to have their entire organization approaching ethical decision making based on the ethical code of the business. For this reason, it is helpful to have the code in writing.

Having a written code of ethics is no guarantee of ethical conduct. Everyone must first understand it, and this will involve training and discussion, which can be part of ongoing employee-development programs. Because some employees will tend to emulate the behavior of managers, regardless of a written code, it is especially critical that people in leadership positions in an organization adhere to ethical standards. The leaders in an organization are not always all managers, so providing training and development in this area is critical.

Ethical dilemmas may arise in just about any situation. Since it is impossible to predict them all, management must stress that ethical behavior is expected, be open to discussion, and be prepared to participate in resolving dilemmas.

Consider an example of the effects of ethical dilemmas and value conflicts on total quality management. As a manager, you must be aware of ways in which conflicts between value systems create ethical dilemmas for clinicians. Some hygienists simply could not ethically accept a client's decision to get full dentures to cure periodontal disease and so would never be happy in a client-driven practice. They would always be under stress caused by providing care they deem ethically unacceptable.

There are numbers of ways to resolve ethical conflicts. For example, an issue may come to light during the strategic planning process, especially when looking at the practice mission and goals, but also when objectives related to quality assurance are discussed. If value conflicts or significant differences in practice philosophies become apparent, they must be resolved, through discussion, workshops, seminars, and the like. Employees who cannot accept the overall plan and practice philosophy will have to be replaced. Employers who wish to keep the best will have to find ways to accept employees' values and judgments, give them decision-making ability, and let them do their jobs their own way.

## Summary

Current concepts in managing for quality include quality control, quality assurance, total quality management, total customer responsiveness, and customer-driven organization. These models emphasize the establishment of client-oriented quality standards, which can be used for continual evaluations of the structure, process, and outcomes of work.

Quality is an issue that will not go away. No manager in any business can afford to avoid issues of quality assurance, standards, and accountability. There are no universal quality standards or applicable mechanisms for any industry, and healthcare delivery is no exception. Healthcare providers face additional ethical challenges in performing their job functions. Their decisions about quality of care affect more than just nuts and bolts but instead may directly and immediately affect peoples lives. Managers and business owners cannot wait for outside authorities to create and impose quality guidelines or ethical standards. They must work within their own organizations to establish internal quality standards and ethical guidelines.

## *Review Questions*

1. Define quality control, quality assurance, quality circle, and total quality management.

2. Discuss the client's role in total quality management of oral healthcare delivery.

3. Give three examples of total quality management of oral healthcare delivery in action.

4. Define the three types of quality assurance standards.

5. Describe an evaluation mechanism for each of the three types of quality assurance standards.

6. Discuss the pros and cons of each mechanism described in Question 5.

7. Describe how a code of ethics might be used in business.

8. Discuss an example of a manager's role in resolving an ethical dilemma.

9. Describe three mechanisms of quality assurance that might be used in dental hygiene practice.

Resolving ethical dilemmas takes practice. There are no right or wrong answers. The following questions are group exercises. Practice role playing in resolving each of the dilemmas presented. Change roles and repeat the process.

10. A dental hygiene client who has a heart murmur and requires antibiotic premedication prior to hygiene treatment comes in for a maintenance visit. The client refuses to take the premedication. She has never actually taken it in the past and nothing has happened. She is willing to sign a statement saying that she has been informed of the risks and refuses to take the antibiotics. The hygienist refuses to treat the client. The dentist-owner insists that the hygienist should treat the client. The office manager, who has recently been to a CE course on risk management, knows that the client's signed statement is not a strong defense against a malpractice suit because the practitioners are legally responsible for providing proper care and they know the client needs the premedication.

11. A client in a periodontal practice requests nitrous oxide for initial therapy (quadrant scaling and root planing) appointments. In this practice, the hygienist provides the initial therapy. The practice is located in a state that does not permit hygienists to administer nitrous oxide. Many patients have made this request. The office manager would like to accommodate their request for their pain control method of choice.

12. In the examples in Questions 10 and 11, what could have been done to prevent these conflicts from surfacing when the patients were present?

13. In countless other areas, conflicts of quality standards and ethics may arise. Some of the common issues involved are infection control, sexual harassment, and assignment/performance of illegal procedures. Using examples from your life, role play the resolution of these conflicts.

## SUGGESTED READING

Cianflone, D., & Riccelli, A. E. (1991). Ethical considerations for dental hygienists in private practice settings. *Journal of Dental Hygiene*, 65(6), 277–279.

Klyop, J. S. (1989). Focusing on quality assurance—The profession's collective efforts. *Journal of Dental Education*, 53(11), 677–678.

Peters, T. (1987). *Thriving on chaos.* New York: HarperCollins.

## REFERENCES

American Dental Association. (1991). *Principles of ethics and code of professional conduct.* Chicago: ADA.

American Dental Hygienists' Association. (1992). *Principles of ethics.* Chicago: ADHA.

American Dental Hygienists' Association. (1993). *Quality assurance and its applications to the delivery of services provided by dental hygienists.* Chicago: ADHA.

Maryniuk, G. A. (1989). Quality assurance: Moving toward implementation. *Journal of Dental Education*, 53(11), 681–682.

Morris, A. L., et al. (1989). The impact of a quality assessment program on the practice behavior of general practitioners: A follow-up study. *Journal of the American Dental Association*, 119, 705–709.

Port, O., and Smith, G. (1992). Quality. *Business Week*, November 30, 1992, pp. 66–75.

# PART 2

# PRACTICE MANAGEMENT

---

*Part 1 covered general principles of business management and some commonly used business terms to provide a basis for discussing the specifics of managing oral health-care delivery presented in this part and other management roles covered in Part 3. Here we will focus on managing clinical practice, in its many different forms.*

*Better management can increase access to care by improving professional and staff relations, by realizing benefits of economy of scale, and by creating new businesses, new jobs, and new roles for dental hygienists. Even if you are not currently employed in a management role, the chapters in this part can provide you with valuable information. If you manage no one but yourself, an increased understanding of oral healthcare delivery from a management perspective can help you improve the quality of care you are able to provide.*

# CHAPTER 6

# The Dental Hygiene Profit Center Defined

## Objectives

After reading this chapter and completing the review questions, the reader should be able to:

- Define profit center.
- Define the dental hygiene profit center.
- Discuss three examples of dental hygiene profit centers.
- Describe the planning function within one type of dental hygiene profit center.
- Describe human resource management within one type of dental hygiene profit center.
- Describe financial management within one type of dental hygiene profit center.
- Describe marketing within one type of dental hygiene profit center.

Dental hygienists are in the best position to understand the management of dental hygiene practice. Better management can increase access to care by improving professional and staff relations, by realizing benefits of economy of scale, and by creating new businesses, new jobs, and new roles for dental hygienists.

Even if you are not currently employed in a management role, Part 2 can provide you with valuable information. If you manage no one but yourself, an increased understanding of dental hygiene practice from a management perspective can help you improve the quality of care you are able to provide. Management functions are similar in dental practice and in dental hygiene practice, but not identical. Many topics covered in Part 2 can be applied to either setting.

## WHAT IS THE DENTAL HYGIENE PROFIT CENTER?

A profit center is a business, or part of a business, operated for profit. A nonprofit business might have profit centers, but they would be operated to break even or to contribute income to some other part of the nonprofit corporation.

Let's consider some examples. If you own a restaurant, that restaurant is operated as a profit center by selling food and beverages. Now consider a chain of fast-food restaurants. All the restaurants in the chain would probably share some operations, such as a distribution network, sources of supply, and advertising costs. Each restaurant in the chain could be managed as a separate profit center with its own share of expenses, for food, supplies, and labor, for example, and its share of profits, from sales. Although some of the expenses might actually be shared (you would purchase hamburger for all the restaurants at the same time to take advantage of quantity discounts), each location would have its own operations. Some locations would be more profitable than others, and the profitability of each could be evaluated separately.

If one corporation owned all the restaurants, there would be one set of financial statements for the corporation as a whole, but each restaurant would also keep its own financial records. In this way, the management of the corporation could see how each location was faring. If all the restaurants were lumped together financially, it would be difficult to understand which locations were prosperous and which were not. By considering each restaurant as a separate profit center, you would be able to analyze the operations of each independently. For example, if, in reviewing the corporate financial statements, you found that you were losing money, you would need to analyze your restaurant operations to find out why and where. By operating each restaurant as a separate profit center, you could examine the records of each location. If you found that only one or two restaurants were losing money, you would then have a starting point for correcting the problem. There is, of course, the possibility that they are losing money equally, and then your problem would be more complicated. At least you would know that some factor common to all locations, such as market segment, price, or distribution, was probably part of the problem.

In many cases the separate profit centers are not so readily identifiable as in the example of the different restaurant locations, and dental hygiene practice falls into this category. Before discussing the dental hygiene profit center, let's look at one more example from a related industry—a large hospital. Within a large hospital are found many different departments, many of them interrelated and not constituted as separate profit centers. For example, because the nursing department probably interfaces with most of the other departments, it would be impossible to consider the nursing department as a separate profit center. Nurses work in intensive care, surgery, and various outpatient clinics, to name just a few, and so function in many different profit centers.

Think of the hospital's functions in terms of centers where clients enter and exit—such as intensive care, the oncology outpatient clinic, and radiology. Each of these functions can be considered as separate profit centers whose income and expenses can be identified. Therefore the overall operation of the hospital can be divided into different profit centers. Once again, this simplifies the management task of analyzing the financial condition of the hospital. This might also be a way to divide management responsibilities, splitting them among the various profit centers. In this way, each management team could stay closely in touch with the profit center for which they are responsible, rather than dividing attention and resources between many different departments. There will, of course, need to be some management of hospital operations as a whole, and, as discussed in Part 1, there are pitfalls to avoid in creating many layers of management.

Because dental hygiene practice and dental practice are closely related, dental hygiene frequently is not regarded as a separate profit center. But, just as within a hospital, where the responsibilities of various departments overlap, there can be significant management advantages to considering dental hygiene practice as a separate profit center. It certainly serves to simplify the discussion of dental hygiene operations.

A dental hygiene profit center (DHPC) is a unit of operations where dental hygiene services are provided. As discussed in the next section, the DHPC can be located in a private dental practice; in a larger, clinical setting, such as a hospital, public health facility, long-term care facility, or in a mobile unit. Most commonly, the DHPC is operated as an integral part of a dental practice. Within any of these practice settings, or others, the DHPC may have any number of financial arrangements.

We will consider some of these arrangements in this chapter. The important point is that management of the DHPC will be considered separately from other profit centers with which it may be involved. Keep in mind that we are discussing business management, not client management. Most states, in their dental practice acts, limit the scope and independence of dental hygiene practice with respect to patient care. The state and federal regulations that pertain to business management are entirely different. Even dental hygiene care delivered in a state with severely restricted dental hygiene practice can still be managed as a dental hygiene profit center. It is a matter of internal financial records, job descriptions, and management decisions, not of supervising client care or of who is present during treatment procedures.

What separates one profit center from another? Mostly, it's just a matter of perspective. In the example of the chain of restaurants, you could look at the controlling corporation as one whole profit center, or look at each restaurant individually. Similarly, a dental group could own several practices in different locations and regard each as separate profit centers. One multispecialty practice, with only one location, could also be divided into separate profit centers, as in the hospital example. The profit centers within such a group might be oral surgery, periodontics, dental hygiene, orthodontics, and dental laboratory. These profit centers might share supplies, administrative or even clinical personnel, and a facility, and each profit center would be assigned a portion of the practice income and expenses. In this way, each could be regarded as a separate profit center within the practice as a whole.

Even a small dental practice might have two or three profit centers, for example, dentistry (restorative, crown and bridge, etc.), surgery (perio, extractions, etc.), and dental hygiene. Each of these profit centers would generate income and expenses. In a small practice there would be a great deal of personnel and management overlap. The following discussion will examine various models for DHPCs.

# TRADITIONAL SETTINGS

By far, the most common setting for most DHPCs is within the private dental practice. Nontraditional settings can be broadly defined as all other settings. Some practice settings, such as clinics within dental or dental hygiene schools, might fall into either category (Schwarz and Mescher, 1989).

The definition of dental hygiene practice varies according to whom you ask, is influenced by state practice acts, and therefore differs from state to state. The definition may also vary from practice to practice, the focus or specialty of the practice, and the clinicians involved. Within any given practice setting, then, the exact definition of the DHPC can be adapted to suit the situation.

The resources of the DHPC will include at least one hygienist. (The maximum number of hygienists employed in one practice is limited in some states.) The DHPC may also include, full time or part time, assistants, dentists, receptionists, bookkeepers, or other administrative personnel, as well as treatment rooms, equipment, instruments, and supplies. The expenses of the DHPC will be incurred for personnel, equipment, supplies, rent, utilities and related costs, and administrative expenses. Sources of income will be services rendered and products sold. These elements will combine to define the DHPC within a private dental practice.

## Dental Practice

It is common to treat dental hygiene practice as part of the dental practice as a whole. As shown in the preceding examples, this merging of profit centers may make it difficult to analyze and manage exactly what is going on within any one.

Consider as an example the following two management approaches. You are the dental practice manager. While reviewing the financial statements for the dental practice you manage, you notice that your operating income margin is falling off. The operating income margin is a profitability ratio, defined as operating earnings divided by income from services. (See Chapter 3 for a discussion of ratios.) After investigating, you decide that this decline is an indication that your operating expenses are too high. You have not treated dental hygiene services as a separate profit center, so you do not have a specific breakdown of income and expenses for dental hygiene. At this point, you cannot document whether the excessive operating expenses are being generated from dental treatment or dental hygiene treatment, or both, confounding your efforts to correct the problem.

Since you lack information about the different profit centers, you take a guess at the problem. Your best guess is that the problem was created by having too many dental hygienists on staff, so you fire two. In the short run, this decreases your operating expenses, but creates new problems. By firing two hygienists, you have significantly reduced the practice income, thrown your recall system into chaos, and created a marketing problem when clients loyal to the two fired hygienists leave your practice. Meanwhile, the other profit centers are still suffering from high operating expenses but it may not become apparent for some time because the overall operating expenses for the practice went down when you fired two hygienists. The other profit centers still have the underlying problem.

While there are times when an informed guess is your only option, your chances of success will be improved if you can base your decisions on actual data. Now suppose you do have data on the DHPC. You review the records for all the profit centers within the practice and compare the profitability ratios for each. Your analysis shows that the problem of increased operating expenses is common to all profit centers. This gives you more information concerning the problem with operating expenses. You can begin by looking for some common problem among them. You find that your health insurance plan has doubled its premiums in the past year. This increase, coupled with hiring two new employees, has caused the increase in operating expenses. This, then, would help you decide how to proceed. You can search for ways to decrease the cost of benefits, or might reassign staff time within the practice to increase profit.

If you found that only the DHPC had a problem with excess operating expenses, you would know that to correct the problem you would have to find a way to decrease operating expenses in the DHPC. If this were the case, you might indeed have reason to fire two hygienists or renegotiate their compensation packages. Having records for the DHPC simplifies this analysis.

When comparing profit centers, compare the ratios. It is important to remember that you can't just compare the operating expenses of each profit center. Some will always be more profitable than others, since many dental procedures are more profitable than dental hygiene procedures. First of all, right or wrong, dentists' time is usually more highly valued than dental hygienists' time, and people are often willing to pay more for time spent with a professional they perceive is more highly trained or has more expertise. Additionally, there is more room for profit margin in dental procedures. Clients don't know how much the dental lab charges for making bridges, only the fee for the entire procedure for preparing and placing the bridge, so the practice can include all of its operating costs in the fee, including dentist time, staff time, lab fees, supplies, and so on. Dental hygienists provide services for which the public generally expects to pay less, partly because clients perceive that they are getting only time with the hygienist, not products, like gold bridgework.

Don't overlook the role that third-party payers (usually insurance companies) play in the value game. They are also willing to pay more for dental treatment, such as crowns, than for preventive visits, the specialty of dental hygienists. Whatever your value judgments may be, the difference in profitability between dental services and dental hygiene services is usually a business fact you must manage. Chapter 8 discusses profitability of the DHPC in more detail.

Considering the DHPC separately from the dental practice makes sense for many reasons. It is sound business practice to do so, even if it is not traditional for the industry. The sources of income for dental practices are limited, as they are for any service sector business. Other than some income, probably a small portion (if any) of the total, generated from product sales, practice income will come from dental services and from dental hygiene services and that's about all. The income, expenses, and profit associated with dental hygiene services will differ from those associated with dental services. As discussed earlier, dental hygiene services are usually less profitable. This does not mean that there is less health value in dental hygiene services. In fact, you could argue that there is more health value in prevention. It does mean that the DHPC will be less profitable than the dental profit center. If you lump the two together, the dental profit center will seem less profitable than it really is and the DHPC will seem more profitable than it really is. Misconception is the mother of mismanagement.

Since we know that the DHPC will usually be less profitable than the dental profit center, let's consider them separately and each on their own merits. The only way to get an accurate picture of either profit center is to separate them. How do you do this? It will take planning and you will need to consult with your accountant. Basically, you make the DHPC a separate business within the business for management purposes. Like the restaurant chain or hospital examples, the DHPC will have overlap with the dental practice.

The DHPC will need management, for planning, for human resources, for finance, and for marketing. Avoid creating too many management layers. The average dental practice that employs dental hygienists employs one dental hygienist (ADA, 1990). Three levels of management are not required. One hygienist can probably manage his clinical duties and manage the DHPC. Another alternative is to have the office manager handle all the profit centers in the practice. Looking at the DHPC separately from the dental practice is more a matter of perspective and record keeping than of meetings and organizational charts.

The DHPC will have costs associated with staff (human resources), administration, equipment and supplies, and marketing. In the DHPC that is part of a dental practice, most of the expenses will be shared with the dental practice. The first step is to review existing financial records and gather any background information on the history of income and expenses for the DHPC. You may find that recordkeeping procedures have to be modified in order to separate the necessary information. After you have sufficient information about the income and expenses for the DHPC and the other profit centers within the practice to analyze or make an intelligent guess, assign portions of the income and expenses to the DHPC and portions to the other profit center(s) within the practice. The secret to success will lie in assigning the correct portions to each. Human resources, finance, and marketing are discussed in more detail in Chapters 7–10.

This will create the DHPC on paper and provide the necessary information to analyze the financial functions of the DHPC separately from the practice of which it is a part. Whether you choose to separate the other management functions of the DHPC will depend on the goals and objectives of the practice. Once you have created the DHPC within the practice, you will be able to fine-tune the operations of the DHPC in accordance with your strategic plan. Notice that in this model of the DHPC within the private dental practice, we have not discussed separating the DHPC from the practice in terms of client management or actual cash flow. We have only changed the record-keeping, paper flow, and management perspective. A client visiting the practice would probably not be aware of these changes. What can change is that better management can lead to improved quality or productivity, again, depending on the goals and objectives of the practice.

## New Dental Hygiene Profit Center

How do you go about starting a DHPC in a traditional setting when none has existed before, in a practice that has never employed a dental hygienist? Begin with the strategic plan. What are the mission and goals of the practice? Does it need a DHPC? Can it supply the necessary resources to start one? If the answers to these questions are yes, develop a strategic plan for the DHPC.

Much of the plan for a start-up operation will involve resource allocation. Where will the financing come from and where will the money go? Briefly, these are the resources the DHPC will need—equipment, supplies, space, employees, and, most importantly, a market for its services. Most of the details of managing these resources are discussed throughout Part 2.

Starting a new DHPC in a nontraditional setting will be similar to a traditional setting. Start with a detailed plan. Most of the same resources will be required, but major differences may exist in funding sources and market base. Finances are considerably different in different practice settings. A new DHPC in an existing dental practice has some existing client pool to draw from, whereas marketing a new DHPC in a new practice setting can be more challenging because a client pool does not exist. Market research must come early in the planning stages to determine whether there even is a market for a DHPC.

## Independent Contracting

In 1980 Linda Kroll published a landmark book on dental hygiene independent contracting, and much has been said and written about this topic since then. What is independent contracting? It is a financial arrangement whereby the dental hygienist is paid as a business operator, not as an employee. The hygienist is not paid a salary by a dental practice. He is paid by the practice for the services he provides. Out of that income, he pays his operating costs, including rent, supplies, equipment, and salary. Notice that this looks like, and is, a DHPC. The difference between independent contracting and the first model of private dental practice is that the DHPC *is* financially independent from the dental practice.

The independent DHPC contracts with dental practices to provide dental hygiene services. The practices pay for this service and the DHPC pays the expenses. Most DHPCs operated under independent contract are closely associated with one dental practice, unless they are independent dental hygiene practices (discussed in the next section). Rather than having an entirely separate facility, the DHPC may be renting space, say one or two treatment rooms, from the dental practice. Staff time, for reception, assisting, or other administrative duties, may also be shared. Equipment and supplies for the DHPC may be purchased from distributors by the DHPC or may be purchased from the dental practice. What makes the DHPC an independent contract arrangement is that the DHPC actually pays for all the operating expenses, even if it is paying the dental practice.

The DHPC operating under independent contracting may be a sole proprietorship (owned by one person), a partnership, or a corporation. In most states this type of business would not be eligible to become a professional association.

Hygienists employed as independent contractors do not receive a salary from any dental practice with which they are associated. No income taxes, social security, or other payroll taxes are withheld. The independent contractors pay the taxes themselves, according to the business structure they have established (different tax laws apply to proprietorships, partnerships, and corporations).

An independent contractor establishes a business relationship with a dental practice (possibly more than one) by verbal or written contract. It is best to have a written contract, developed with the help of an attorney, containing all the specifics of how income and expenses are to be handled. If you have little or no experience in this area, help from an attorney is a necessity. Contract completion will be expedited if you develop your strategic plan and write down your specific requirements for receiving payments and meeting expenses before meeting with the attorney to discuss the first draft of the contract. You may begin negotiations with the dental practice before you draft the contract, or you may prepare the first draft ahead of time and then negotiate.

There are specific Internal Revenue Service (IRS) requirements regarding independent contracting. They change periodically, and you must consult with an accountant knowledgeable in this area before establishing yourself as an independent contractor. In general, the IRS stipulates that independent contractors set their own hours, purchase their own equipment and supplies, and collect their own payments for services. Failure to comply with the IRS requirements can have serious consequences. As an independent contractor, you pay taxes differently than you would as an employee. If you file your taxes as an independent contractor and the IRS disallows your independent contractor status (says that you do not meet its requirements), you will probably have a major tax problem and may be liable for significant penalties for misfiling. If you owe significantly more taxes than you have paid, you will be liable to pay the correct tax, plus interest and penalties on the amount of unpaid taxes. Do not practice as an independent contractor without getting advice from the IRS or knowledgeable attorneys or accountants in advance. Be sure that you understand what taxes to pay and when, where, and how to pay them. If you get into trouble with the IRS, it can affect your income for years.

Payment for dental hygiene services can be an issue for independent contractors. Most insurance companies will not pay a dental hygienist for dental hygiene services unless the hygienist is an independent practitioner. Insurance payments for preventive oral healthcare usually only go to dentists. Dental hygienists are not direct healthcare providers unless they work without supervision (there are exceptions to this). What this means for the DHPC operated under an independent contract is that it will rarely be able to collect payments directly from insurance companies. Clients with insurance will have to pay the DHPC in cash or direct the insurance payment to the associated dental practice, and the DHPC will then have to collect the money from the dental practice. As a result, clients with insurance may choose to receive care at a DHPC that does accept insurance (one that is part of a dental practice).

As the healthcare delivery system has changed and more allied health professionals have become direct care providers, insurance companies have been obliged to pay them. The insurance industry has strongly resisted this trend because of its potential to generate significantly more paid claims, which may amount to billions of dollars within the entire insurance industry. While clients seeking care from these providers would probably have gotten it regardless of where the insurance payment went, insurance companies have been reluctant to see it this way.

An alternative to collecting payments directly from clients would be to have the dental practice(s) you are working with collect payments. The practice would then pay you fees according to your contract with the practice, and you would avoid the direct costs for labor and supplies for billing, insurance processing, and collections. These costs would be passed on indirectly from the dental practice, again according to your contract with the practice. As with any business negotiations, there are many possible variations on payment arrangements and so the exact terms for each DHPC operating under independent contract would vary from case to case.

Restrictions on dental hygiene practice vary from state to state and can be considerable. You must be familiar with your state practice act and the rules and regulations established by the state licensing board. Independent contracting is a business arrangement. It is not directly related to supervision requirements, but, of course, supervision requirements will affect the way you practice.

If you practice in a state that requires that a dentist be physically present in the facility during dental hygiene treatment, the hours you will be able to practice will be limited, but, as an independent contractor you will be able to vary your hours within these limits. You may also be able to contract with dentists to provide supervision for the DHPC during the hours you prefer.

If you practice in a state that requires that dental hygiene clients be clients of record of a dentist, or that you work with a dentist's prescription for treatment, you will need to document, for each client, that you have complied with these rules. Furthermore, there may be many other rules and regulations that you must obey. Be sure you are familiar with all the pertinent laws, rules, and regulations and that you carefully document that you have complied with them. All of these factors, as well as the political climate, must be considered in the development of the strategic plan for the DHPC.

Linda Kroll encountered significant opposition from organized dentistry when she first became an independent contractor. There are significant costs associated with this type of lengthy legal struggle. Since the first test cases, some dental hygiene independent contractors have not had substantial legal or political problems, but others have. You will need to estimate your risks and costs in the early planning stages. Working with your state and local dental hygiene association is the best place to begin your assessment. The dental hygiene association may provide your strongest base of support.

Independent contractors may be found in many different practice settings, including private dental practice, mobile clinics, public health facilities, long-term care facilities, hospitals, or prisons. Whether it is possible to work as an independent contractor in any of these settings in a particular state will partly depend on the practice act. The deciding factor may be the negotiating skills of the independent contractor. If he is able to persuade others to pay for his services as an independent contractor, the other obstacles can be overcome.

What remains is the question of profitability. Not all DHPCs can succeed operating as independent contract arrangements. Careful analysis and planning are necessary before establishing the independent contract DHPC. If, in developing a realistic business plan, you discover that you cannot succeed as an independent contractor in a given location or market, you will have to either change your plan (i.e., choose a new location or market) or give up the idea.

# NONTRADITIONAL SETTINGS

The preceding discussion focused on DHPCs in the traditional private practice setting. DHPCs exist in nontraditional settings as well, including unsupervised practice, schools, hospitals, with or without dental clinics, various types of public health facilities, both public and private long-term care facilities, and mobile clinics. Estimates of the number of dental hygienists practicing in nontraditional settings range from 5% to 11.8% (Schwarz & Mescher, 1989).

There are additional models of dental hygiene practice not discussed in detail here. The entire healthcare delivery system is changing. As this trend continues, new opportunities will probably be created for nontraditional dental hygiene practice. The common denominator among these practice settings is the provision of dental hygiene services, with associated income and expenses. Each of these settings is an example of a DHPC in operation. From a business perspective, much of what goes on in any practice setting will be similar, even if the modes of treatment delivery vary. The following discussion of non-traditional dental hygiene practice focuses on management operations that are likely to change in different settings.

## Unsupervised Practice

As of the publication date of this book, unsupervised practice is legal only in Colorado and in some practice settings in Washington, though several other states are pursuing it. Unsupervised practice is often referred to as independent practice, although this terminology often confuses unsupervised practice with independent contracting. The two are not the same. As already discussed, it is possible to work as an independent contractor, regardless of supervision requirements. An unsupervised dental hygiene practice is a DHPC that is not linked with any particular dental practice. The dental hygienists working without supervision are not required to have a dentist physically present in the facility during dental hygiene treatment, are not required to see clients of record of a dentist, and do not require a dentist's prescription for treatment.

From a business standpoint, an unsupervised dental hygiene practice might look very much like other DHPCs, except that it would not be required to have the services of a dentist, thereby eliminating the associated costs. An unsupervised practice might, of course, choose to employ or contract with dentists and would then incur these costs. Most states restrict who can own a dental practice and/or dental equipment, so these laws would have a significant impact on an unsupervised DHPC.

Like the DHPC that operated under independent contract, the owners of an unsupervised dental hygiene practice would assume considerable financial risk, as do the owners of a dental practice. Income and expenses would be comparable with similar DHPCs operating in analogous markets. At the present time, malpractice insurance rates are the same for independent contractors and unsupervised practitioners, and slightly higher than those of dental hygienists practicing as employees. All of the discussion in Part 2 would be equally applicable to any DHPC, regardless of supervision requirements.

## The School Setting

School settings may encompass a variety of choices. DHPCs may be located in or associated with dental or dental hygiene schools or elementary through high schools. Some public school settings are part of public health programs, and so management factors of both school and public health settings will be involved.

Planning for school settings can be considerably more complicated than it is for traditional settings. The manager of the DHPC has much less input into management decisions of the school setting as a whole and therefore has to adapt planning for the DHPC to the planning methods used by the school. There are likely to be more layers of management involved, as well as more political involvement, both internal and external, in the planning process. The budgeting cycle may not be closely related to other parts of strategic planning, so the manager of the DHPC may have to develop a slightly different strategic planning model than the one discussed in Chapter 1.

The personnel policies of the DHPC in a school probably conform to those of the school or public health agency controlling the DHPC. Due to budget limitations, the staff of the school-based DHPC is probably quite small, maybe just one or two people. As part of a small business, the DHPC within a private dental practice may be exempt from some laws or government rules and regulations, such as provisions of the Americans with Disabilities Act. DHPCs located in public facilities, such as schools, however, may have to comply with all of these requirements, as the schools must, to qualify for government funds.

The finances of the DHPC are closely linked with those of the controlling organization. A DHPC within a school is probably part of a not-for-profit organization, and as such the planning and financial goals of the DHPC will differ. The manager of the DHPC may have limited input into financial decisions that affect the DHPC, but he can take steps to maximize the effectiveness of his input. The first of these is to keep financial records for the DHPC, even if this is not required, so that the manager has accurate income and expense information available at all times. Second, being knowledgeable about the finances of the controlling organization and its budgeting process will help the DHPC manager anticipate the financial climate within the organization, plan effectively for the DHPC, and justify any financial suggestions made during the budgeting process. Finally, finances within public settings are likely to be influenced by politics. The manager who understands the political situation and how to work within it will increase the likelihood of success for the DHPC.

The need for marketing for the school-based DHPC may be limited. If it has a predefined market of students, there won't be a need for advertising or sales. The public relations efforts of the school-based DHPC would revolve around community involvement. The greatest potential for utilizing marketing skills would probably be in the area of delivering effective public health and disease prevention messages to the population served by the DHPC.

## The Hospital Setting

Because most hospitals receive at least part of their funding from government sources, they, like schools, are affected by extensive government rules and regulations and also by politics. Additionally, most hospitals are large, complex organizations. The DHPC within a hospital setting probably has fewer than 20 employees and operates internally like a small business. Being part of the hospital, however, the DHPC must comply with many of the requirements affecting large businesses and may have some of the same problems.

The DHPC may have its own internal planning system. The manager will have to integrate DHPC operations with the planning cycle of the hospital. This will be especially critical with regard to budget planning.

Human resource management within the hospital-based DHPC will also be affected by government requirements pertaining to the hospital, especially if the DHPC or the department of which it is a part is receiving any government funding. For example, provisions of the Americans with Disabilities Act not affecting small business would probably apply to the DHPC that is part of a hospital. Complying with these requirements can be quite costly. This should be taken into account during budget planning, especially for a start-up (new) DHPC.

The DHPC within a hospital may have human resources available to it that a private practice would not. The DHPC would probably have greater access to medical and nursing expertise, which can be important to the hospital-based DHPC because hospitalized clients have more medical needs than do ambulatory clients. Additionally, volunteer help might be available, either through the hospital or through associated professional schools of nursing, dental hygiene, or dentistry. Participating in such programs is a community service and can offer the DHPC significant cost savings.

The complexity of finances within the DHPC will be related to the complexity of the hospital. The effects may be less noticeable if the DHPC is operated as an independent contract arrangement. Hospitals may be for-profit or non-for-profit and the profit orientation of the hospital is reflected in most of its management functions.

The DHPC will probably be a part of some other department within the hospital, for example, the dental clinic. As with the case of the school-based DHPC, it will be advantageous for the DHPC to maintain its own financial records whenever possible. This will facilitate management of the DHPC, provide management with up-to-the-minute information when needed, and provide backup for funding requests. Additional funding sources may be available to the hospital-based DHPC, such as grants from charitable foundations or research grants. Finding such sources may require a bit of investigation, but it may be worth the effort.

The marketing efforts of the DHPC will be influenced by the profit orientation of the hospital as well. Hospitals do advertise, sometimes for specific services they offer. The DHPC might be included in some of this advertising. There probably will not be any sales management required. Hospital marketing is frequently centered on public relations and community service and there is plenty of room for DHPC involvement in these efforts.

## Public Health Facilities

Much of the previous discussion about public institutions applies to public health facilities as regards planning, human resources, finance, and politics. The DHPC in a public health setting must comply with many more government requirements than does a small business, both in human resource and client management. Public health facilities, of course, have a not-for-profit orientation. Since the trend toward reduced funding of public health programs is expected to continue for the near future, more funding may have to come from private sources, and the DHPC manager may become a fund-raiser.

There is considerable public debate about the need for national health policy. Under a national health system, government would employ healthcare providers directly and manage the healthcare delivery system. The numbers of private healthcare providers would be greatly reduced. This is the type of system currently used in England. Under a national health insurance system, by contrast, the government would provide only the health insurance. While this plan would not have the same impact on the numbers of private providers that a national health system would, national health insurance would give the federal government considerable control of healthcare costs. If either of these systems are adopted in the United States, it will have a tremendous impact on all types of healthcare delivery, especially on practice within public health settings.

Many states currently have different practice restrictions affecting dental hygiene practice in some public health settings. Some allow for general supervision of hygienists and some allow for unsupervised practice. Differences in state practice acts would affect the operation of the DHPC in a public health setting.

As in the case of the school-based DHPC, marketing efforts on behalf of the DHPC are minimal. Creative marketing energies can be channeled into public health and prevention messages.

## Long-Term Care Facilities

Long-term care facilities are nursing homes and extended-care facilities. Extended-care facilities are a link between the total care provided in a nursing home and out-patient care. As with public health facilities, some states have broader supervision requirements for dental hygiene practice in long-term care facilities.

Client needs within the long-term care facility setting differ from those within the private practice setting. Clients requiring long-term care have more complex medical conditions. Planning for the DHPC must take this into account. The medical needs of clients will require that additional medical and nursing consultations be available, and special equipment, such as mobile hand pieces, will probably be needed. This will affect the financial requirements of the DHPC, and possibly the staffing requirements. As in the case of the hospital-based DHPC, marketing efforts for the DHPC may be linked to those of the long-term care facility and may be limited to public relations activities.

## Mobile Clinics

The mobile DHPC may be an independent dental hygiene practice, or it may be associated with any of the other practice settings discussed previously. The planning, staffing, and financial requirements of the DHPC closely resemble those of the associated practice setting. Additionally, the mobile DHPC may have to comply with government regulations not affecting other practice settings. This varies from state to state. Staffing requirements may be affected. The DHPC will need personnel familiar with or able to be trained on mobile equipment. Provisions will have to be made for driving and equipment maintenance. Mobile clinics may have slightly different funding sources or billing practices.

A common theme for all nontraditional practice settings is that the DHPCs may have nontraditional needs. Your network of professional contacts can be a great source of information regarding the availability of special funding or equipment or human resources. Additionally, the American Dental Hygienists' Association is a valuable source of professional information for dental hygienists in all types of practice settings.

As the healthcare delivery system changes and new practice settings are established, existing networks may not exist for a particular interest group. As a manager of such a practice setting, you may find it helpful to establish some new network, starting with your existing professional affiliations, or those in the practice setting, as a basis for information and contacts.

# THE ACCELERATED DENTAL HYGIENE PRACTICE

Accelerated dental hygiene practice is a term frequently used to describe a DHPC that employs assistants to enable the hygienists to work at an accelerated pace. There are some points to keep in mind when discussing accelerated practice. Oral healthcare delivery involves treating the entire client, not just cleaning teeth. Hygienists and assistants provide comprehensive care for their clients, not just isolated services. It is helpful, however, to consider a list of common procedures that assistants might perform (see Table 6.1). Not all of the procedures listed in the table can legally be performed in every state, but the list may serve as a general guideline for discussion.

In an accelerated dental hygiene practice, assistants are employed to the maximum capacity permitted by law. The hygiene assistants may perform any or all of the services listed in Table 6.1. Multiple treatment rooms are required in the DHPC in order to operate at an accelerated practice. Working with an assistant, and using two or three treatment rooms, one dental hygienist is able to treat more clients than can a single hygienist working alone out of one room.

## Starting an Accelerated Practice—One Example

A dental practice in a rural area experienced a large increase in the number of clients due to the expansion of nearby suburban areas. The practice employed the dentist-owner, a receptionist/bookkeeper, and one dental hygienist. The den-

---

***Table 6.1* • PROCEDURES THAT MAY BE PERFORMED BY HYGIENE ASSISTANTS**

Greet client
Escort client to operatory
Seat client
Assist hygienist during scaling, polishing, or fluoride treatment
Assist hygienist during placement of sealants
Expose x-rays
Process x-rays
Record during periodontal probing
Record during hard tissue charting
Brush or floss client's teeth (plaque removal)
Oral hygiene instructions
Apply topical fluoride
Dismiss client
Operatory maintenance (i.e., infection control procedures)

---

tist-owner acted as practice manager. There were three equipped treatment rooms. As the practice acquired more and more new clients, it became increasingly difficult to get an appointment with the dental hygienist. The new suburban developments had fluoridated water and therefore limited restorative needs, but most of the new clients needed dental hygiene and/or periodontal treatment. Although the dentist had taken many CE courses on periodontics and did provide some advanced periodontal treatment, he didn't have time in his schedule to treat all the initial therapy clients. The practice needed to expand its ability to treat the periodontal and general maintenance clients, as well as to provide initial evaluations for all the new clients.

The increased client pool had generated sufficient income to allow the practice to equip a fourth operatory. In this rural area, however, there were few dental hygienists looking for jobs and the owner was unable to find a hygienist who was right for the practice. In the search, however, the owner and staff did encounter several assistants who seemed right for the practice. They decided to create a separate DHPC to operate as an accelerated hygiene practice, and the dental hygienist who had been with the practice for several years became the DHPC manager. He continued his clinical duties as well, with additional time added to his schedule to complete his management tasks.

The DHPC manager decided to hire one of the assistants identified earlier. The assistant was a certified dental assistant (CDA) with experience in taking radiographs and giving client instructions. He seemed to believe in the mission of the practice and was interested in becoming a dental hygiene assistant. The assistant joined the practice and began working with the hygienist, learning the operation of the DHPC. As part of the office's ongoing training program, the entire staff went to several CE courses, sponsored by the state dental hygiene association, which emphasized dental hygiene practice. This helped to prepare everyone in the group to gear up for supporting the new accelerated hygiene practice.

In the beginning, the hygiene schedule was not changed. Clients continued to receive the same length appointments that they had in the past. The assistant performed duties in the DHPC similar to those he had performed as a dental assistant—infection control procedures, greeting and dismissing clients, taking and processing radiographs. The hygienist and assistant began to use both treatment rooms to increase their work efficiency. If clients came in early or late or needed additional time to meet with the dentist, they were able to use the second treatment room.

The strategic plan for the DHPC called for implementing the full-scale accelerated practice six months after the start-up date. As hygiene clients scheduled their six-month maintenance appointments, the receptionist scheduled them into the accelerated plan with one-hour appointments, unless the hygienist indicated that some variation was needed. The clients were scheduled at half-hour intervals, so that one client arrived every 30 minutes for a one-hour appointment.

By the time the six-month deadline arrived, the assistant was fully trained in his duties as hygiene assistant and the hygienist had learned to work smoothly with assistance. The receptionist was completely familiar with the scheduling scheme and all the insurance codes for DHPC procedures.

This is how operations usually proceeded in the DHPC. The assistant seated the first client, updated the client's health history, took a blood pressure measurement, opened all the sterile instrument packs, and put out fresh disposables. The assistant reviewed and noted the client's chief complaint and reviewed the oral hygiene instructions from the last visit. This took the first 15 minutes of the client's appointment. The hygienist would then come in and perform his assessment. If he identified a need for radiographs, the assistant took them if he was free or the hygienist took them and left them for the assistant to process. The hygienist then completed his plan and treated the client, including giving any new home care instructions and making his notes in the chart.

In the meantime, the assistant had 15 minutes before the next client arrived to complete any necessary cleaning or preparations in the second treatment room or to take or process radiographs, if needed, or to assist the hygienist in charting. At 30 minutes after the hour, the second client arrived, and the assistant then spent 15 minutes on the same initial tasks he performed with the first client.

At the end of the 15 minutes, the hygienist had completed his work with the first client. The assistant then returned to the first client to assist the dentist in his examination of the client. When the examination was complete, the assistant accompanied the client to the receptionist's desk, thanked the client for coming in, and gave the receptionist the routing slip and any special instructions for reappointing the client. The assistant was also available to ask the hygienist or dentist any last-minute questions from the client, or to answer them himself. The assistant then had time to complete infection control procedures in the first treatment room and set up for the third client. Meanwhile, the hygienist finished his work with the second client and the cycle began again.

When the accelerated practice was in full operation, the small, rural dental practice was able to double the number of clients treated in the DHPC. Each client was able to have a one-hour appointment, although children were generally given shorter appointments. Notice that this practice was successful in meeting its clients' increased demand for care without compromising quality and without fill-ing up the dentist's schedule with hygiene clients. The dentist was busy, however, doing exams, treatment planning, and periodontal therapy.

The dentist and hygienist continued their recruitment efforts and networking. If the practice continued to be flooded with new clients, they would be ready to expand the DHPC.

## Income Effects of Accelerated Practice

Compare the case of (1) one hygienist working out of one treatment room to the case of (2) one hygienist and one assistant working out of two treatment rooms. In case 1, if the hygienist treats 8 clients in 8 hours (one hour per client), he will treat 8 clients per day, 40 clients per 5-day workweek, and 2000 clients per 50-week work year. In case 2, if the hygienist spends 30 minutes with each client and the assistant spends 30 minutes with each client (each client still has a one-hour appointment), working on a staggered schedule out of two treatment rooms, the hygienist/assis-tant combination will treat twice as many clients per day and per year—16 versus 8 per day, and 4000 versus 2000 per year.

The income implications are as follows (see Table 6.2). In case 1, if the average case fee is $50, the solo hygienist would generate $100,000 in income per year. In case 2, with the same $50 average case fee, the accelerated practice would generate $200,000 in income per year. A rough estimate of yearly expenses might be that the hygienist earns $40,000 per year, the assistant earns $20,000 per year, and the total of other expenses for the DHPC is 20% of gross income. In case 1, the expenses would be $40,000 for the hygienist plus $20,000 for expenses (20% of $100,000) for a total of $60,000. This would leave a profit margin of 40% and a yearly profit of $40,000. In case 2, the expenses would be $40,000 for the hygienist plus $20,000 for the assistant, plus $40,000 for expenses (20% of $200,000) for a total of $100,000. This would leave a profit margin of 50% and a yearly profit of $100,000.

These estimates are conservative. If, in the overhead expense category, taxes and benefits for the employees were high, or supplies were unusually costly, or if the DHPC had a large debt burden, total overhead might be more than 20%. If the total overhead expenses were 30% (still a reasonable figure), the profit in case

*Table 6. 2 •* **FINANCIAL ESTIMATES FOR TWO DHPCs**

|  | Case 1 | Case 2 |
|---|---|---|
| Income | $100,000 | $200,000 |
| Expenses |  |  |
|   Hygienist | 40,000 | 40,000 |
|   Assistant |  | 20,000 |
|   Overhead | 20,000 | 40,000 |
|   Total | 60,000 | 100,000 |
|   Profit | 40,000 | 100,000 |

1 would be $30,000 and in case 2 $80,000. The profit for the accelerated practice would still be more than double the profit for the solo hygienist.

Beyond financial considerations, accelerated dental hygiene practice offers help for underserved populations. Note that the accelerated DHPC treats twice as many clients as the more traditional DHPC without assistants. In an area where clients are in desperate need of dental hygiene treatment, but hygienists are in short supply, an accelerated practice would double the number of available hygiene appointments. This would depend on the DHPC being able to recruit qualified assistants.

While there are both treatment and financial benefits to accelerated dental hygiene practice, there are some potentially negative aspects to consider. First, there is no published research regarding the quality of care provided in an accelerated practice. In the preceding example, each client had a one-hour appointment—30 minutes with the hygienist and 30 minutes with the assistant. This model assumes that the quality of care received in the 30 minutes with the assistant is equal to the quality of care the client would have received if that 30 minutes had been spent with the hygienist. No doubt, in many cases the quality of care would be equal and it is certainly possible that the management and staff of the DHPC would be sure that it is. The question is raised, however, because hygienists are required to have much more postsecondary education than are assistants and are also licensed. The American Dental Assistants' Association is working hard to establish a national standard for assistants' training, but at this time there is no national standard for all assistants and they are not licensed. In some states, assistants are not regulated at all, and the existing regulations vary widely from state to state.

While the issues of education and regulation are decided in the political arena, what is the manager of the DHPC to do in the meantime? Assure that *every* staff member in the DHPC is educated, well qualified, and has up-to-date training to perform all the duties the job requires.

Another quality issue may be raised by clients themselves. The practice will have to solicit input from clients regarding their feelings about being treated in the accelerated practice. Phobic clients may suffer from increased anxiety when being treated by several different people or if they feel rushed. Some clients may not respond well to being treated by two different individuals in one appointment, especially if they are used to seeing one clinician for the entire appointment. Other clients may not mind or may not even notice. After all, many clients are used to seeing both the hygienist and the dentist in one appointment. If an accelerated practice gives clients a longer appointment for the same price as the short appointment in the traditional DHPC, they may perceive this as an added value. However, some clients may perceive an added value only if they have a longer appointment with one provider. Clients may perceive the change as less time with the dental hygienist, especially if the DHPC changes to accelerated practice without incorporating a change to longer scheduled appointments. These factors will have to be considered in the initial planning for the accelerated practice and evaluated as the changes are implemented.

These are marketing questions that you will have to address before beginning an accelerated practice. Part of the success of the accelerated practice will depend on how it is presented to clients. In the end, some market segments will respond well and others will not. You will have to modify your strategic plan accordingly.

Accelerated dental hygiene practice may present a legal and ethical dilemma for some practitioners. Consumers are not always aware of the education and licensure differences between assistants and hygienists. Many view these roles as interchangeable, although assistants' salaries are usually lower than hygienists' salaries. This combination of facts may create a temptation to ask assistants to perform duties that are illegal, that is, duties that are by statute (law) or by rules and regulations of the dental board to be performed only by hygienists or dentists. Illegal or unethical practice will, in the long run, create negative repercussions for the DHPC (both legal and financial) and must be avoided. It is the manager's responsibility to be sure that operations in the DHPC are conducted in an ethical and responsible manner. (Also see Ethics in Chapter 5.)

Another hazard associated with the accelerated practice is the risk of employee burnout. The success of accelerated practice depends on treating significant numbers of clients in an efficient manner. Each clinician probably has some work load comfort zone, some number of clients he can treat in one day without feeling like part of an assembly line. Not everyone will be comfortable in an accelerated practice, so the DHPC manager will have to recruit those who are.

There are financial risks in establishing an accelerated practice. Each hygienist will need at least two treatment rooms, and there can be considerable cost in expanding office space and equipping each room. If there are no assistants in the DHPC, at least one will have to be hired and trained to create an accelerated practice. The DHPC will have to begin paying the assistant immediately, although the new accelerated practice probably will not generate its total estimated maximum income immediately. This can create a significant cash flow problem. Issues of human resource, financial, and marketing management are addressed in detail in Chapters 7–10.

## Summary

The dental hygiene profit center is a unit of operations that provides dental hygiene services. A DHPC may be located in a traditional, private practice setting or in any number of nontraditional settings. The personnel of the DHPC may be employees, independent contractors, independent practitioners, or some combination of these types. The DHPC can be regarded as a separate unit of operations, regardless of the practice setting or financial arrangements. It is to management's advantage to run the dental hygiene operation as a separate profit center. This will provide management with accurate information with which to make decisions and can be especially useful in planning and evaluation.

## Review Questions

1. Define profit center.
2. Define the dental hygiene profit center.

3. Discuss three examples of dental hygiene profit centers.

4. Describe the planning function within one type of dental hygiene profit center.

5. Describe human resource management within one type of dental hygiene profit center.

6. Describe financial management within one type of dental hygiene profit center.

7. Describe marketing within one type of dental hygiene profit center.

8. Describe the type of dental hygiene profit center that you would most like to manage. Why is this your choice?

9. Write the initial, descriptive section of a business plan for your ideal dental hygiene profit center. Note that you may need to complete studying all of Part 2 before completing the business plan.

## SUGGESTED READING

Basset, L. C., & Metzger, N. (1986). *Achieving excellence: A prescription for healthcare managers.* Rockville: Aspen Publishers.

Gumpert, D. (1990). *How to really create a successful business plan.* Boston: Inc. Publishing.

Longest, B. B. (1990). *Management practices for the health professional.* Norwalk: Appleton and Lange.

Thomas, R. D. (1987). *Career directions for dental hygienists.* New Jersey: Career Directions Press.

Thompson, E. M. (1989). Marketing the dental hygienist as a manager in oral healthcare settings. *Journal of Dental Hygiene,* 63(7), 336–340.

Woodall, I., & Bentley, J. M. (1983). *Legal, ethical, and management aspects of the dental care system* (2nd ed.). St. Louis: C.V. Mosby.

## REFERENCES

American Dental Association. (1990). *Survey of dental practice.* Chicago: ADA.

Kroll, L. (1980). A room with no window. Torrance, Cal.: Author.

Schwarz, I., & Mescher, K. (1989). Office profile. *Journal of Dental Hygiene,* 63(4), 185–190.

# CHAPTER 7

# Managing Human Resources in Oral Healthcare Delivery

---

## Objectives

After reading this chapter and completing the review questions, the reader should be able to:

- Discuss three principles of scientific management and how these relate to dental hygiene or dental practice.
- Compare and contrast Maslow's and Herzberg's theories of motivation.
- Discuss two examples of ways in which planning can impact various practices.
- Describe four methods of compensation.
- List and discuss six key employment issues.
- Discuss the pros and cons of using job descriptions.
- Discuss the pros and cons of using employment contracts.
- Define and discuss the noncompetition clause.
- Discuss the impact of OSHA regulations on oral healthcare delivery.
- List at least six topics to include in a practice procedure manual and state your justification for including them.

---

## MOTIVATION

A number of theories of human resource management, developed in industry, are directly applicable to managing oral healthcare delivery. One of the oldest models, and one that is often followed unconsciously in many practices, is based on the theory of scientific management developed by Taylor (Donnelly, Gibson, & Ivancevich, 1989). Another model, familiar to most dental hygienists, is Maslow's hierarchy of needs (Maslow, 1990). One final model that is relevant to managing oral healthcare delivery is Herzberg's theory of maintenance and motivational factors (Herzberg, 1971). How can these management models be applied to motivating and managing people in oral healthcare delivery?

## Lessons Learned from Scientific Management

In some circles, practice employees are managed as though the provision of health services is a factory operation, churning out treated patients, with each service or procedure a part of a process. Is this an effective method for managing healthcare providers in the twenty-first century? What lessons can the manager learn from the theory of scientific management?

The basic principles of Taylor's theory of scientific management state that management should

1. Plan the work to be done by predetermining the expected quantity and quality of output of each job.
2. Organize the work to be done by specifying the appropriate ways to perform each job.
3. Select and train qualified individuals.
4. Oversee the actual job performance.
5. Verify that actual quantity and quality of output meets expectations.

In other words, management experts can divide every job into tasks that can then be arranged efficiently to produce maximum productivity. All good workers need to achieve maximum productivity is an efficient work plan and careful management. Under a system of scientific management as proposed by Taylor, productivity is linked to financial incentives so that the more the worker produces, the more the worker earns. Management demands for increased productivity are thus satisfied and workers are motivated to produce as much as possible.

Taylor's methods have been applied in many practices, often without success, as evidenced by the conflicts between many assistants, dental hygienists, dentists, and their employers and many declining dental practices. Can we apply the principles of scientific management to dental or dental hygiene practice? Consider the following facts about scientific management. The theory of scientific management, developed by Frederick Taylor in 1911, was based on his observations of manual laborers, most of whom were illiterate, loading heavy chunks of pig iron onto railway cars. Taylor believed that the workers were incapable of designing an efficient work plan on their own and that it was the responsibility of management to tell each worker, in infinite detail, how to complete the work tasks and to supervise their work closely. Most of his theories are no longer accepted management theory because they do not apply to most modern jobs.

Although at first glance the principles of scientific management appear to be applicable to oral healthcare delivery, a closer examination raises some important points. First, clients deserve better care than chunks of iron, and, unlike pieces of iron, they also expect individualized attention. Second, dentists and dental hygienists are licensed, college-educated professionals, not illiterate laborers. They are perfectly capable of, and have years of training in preparation for, planning their own work and client treatment. They do not need managers to give them detailed instructions on task completion or to closely supervise and evaluate their work.

The field of healthcare delivery is complex, detailed, and becoming more so. Delivering professional services in a potentially infectious environment is a job that requires careful education and regulation. That task is not to be equated with shoveling iron by the ton. Consumers expect, and deserve, thoughtful treatment in a safe environment.

## Solutions from Maslow and Herzberg

Chapter 1 included a discussion of Walter Wriston's definition of the manager's role. "The job of the manager today: find the best people you can, motivate them, and allow them to do the job their own way" (Wriston, 1990). An additional implication of this statement is that motivating the best people and allowing them to do their jobs their own way is the best way to get them to stay with you. It is especially true in a service business that the employees are the business. A successful dental hygiene or dental practice depends on clients' trust and confidence in the healthcare providers involved. It makes sense therefore that a practice should hire the best and keep them because so much depends on the clients' rapport with the staff members.

Maslow and Herzberg offer good solutions. Briefly, Maslow's theory, introduced about 1943, is based on his hypothesis of the existence of a hierarchy of needs. He stated that the lower-level needs must be satisfied before a person can deal with the higher-level needs. In his hierarchy, the lower-order needs are the basic physiological human needs (food, water, shelter, sex), safety and stability, and social needs (love, satisfying interpersonal relationships). The higher-order needs are esteem (respect, recognition, self-esteem) and self-actualization (fulfillment of one's personal and creative goals).

For management, the implications of Maslow's theory are that employees' physiological, safety, and social needs must be met before they can focus on issues related to esteem and self-actualization. Employees working to fulfill lower-level needs will tend to require more management and will be more internally focused. Managers need to motivate people toward fulfilling the higher-level needs because employees working at higher levels will be more self-directed, independently productive, and focused on the good of the group (i.e., practice). Managers can help employees satisfy their esteem needs by recognizing outstanding performance and by offering responsibility, authority, and significant work activities. Managers can help employees satisfy their self-actualization needs by offering challenging work and advancement opportunities and by encouraging creativity.

Herzberg's theory, introduced in 1959, divided job conditions into two categories: maintenance factors and motivational factors. Although not strong motivators, the maintenance factors are necessary to sustain a reasonable level of satisfaction. Maintenance factors include work conditions, personal life, job security, salary, interpersonal relationships, and competent technical supervision. The absence of adequate maintenance factors leads to job dissatisfaction, but their presence does not necessarily lead to increased motivation.

Herzberg's motivational factors include achievement, recognition, challenging work, responsibility, and opportunity for personal growth. An absence of these factors does not lead to job dissatisfaction, but their presence can provide strong motivation. For management, the implications of Herzberg's theory are that maintenance factors need to be in place to prevent job dissatisfaction and that motivating factors are necessary to promote outstanding job performance. Furthermore, highly motivated employees tend to have a high tolerance for missing maintenance factors.

Health insurance benefits may be an exception to conventional thinking on needs theory and compensation. Because the cost of health insurance has become quite high, the loss of insurance benefits may pose a threat to employees' lower-level and maintenance needs. An employee who does not have or loses health insurance benefits and is unable to afford or obtain insurance from another source may face a significant personal crisis. While compensation may not be a motivator, it is important to remember that complete absence or loss of some benefits, such as health insurance, can entirely change an employee's focus and, subsequently, job performance.

Managers and business owners are under almost constant pressure to increase profits and decrease expenses. At first glance, the principles of scientific management offer an easy solution, but more than 80 years of research and experience have proven that these principles do not apply to skilled jobs (Donnelly, Gibson, & Ivancevich, 1984). Financial incentives are not highly motivating to people whose basic needs are being met. Both Maslow and Herzberg have demonstrated more effective ways to motivate workers. And while healthcare providers must be productive, they must also be educated and responsible. Prevention of disease transmission is at the core of every health service provided. No amount of productivity can be meaningful if, in the end, the client contracts a debilitating or fatal disease during treatment.

Practice owners and managers must consider that without a market, there is no business. Clients who feel that being treated by unqualified individuals or under unsafe conditions is endangering their health will seek treatment elsewhere. Management expert Tom Peters has pointed out that "in today's market, no point of differentiation is likely to prove more powerful than quality. . . . Quality equals profit" (Peters, 1987). If clients feel they are being hustled through an assembly line in your practice, they will probably seek treatment elsewhere.

A practice must meet the market demand for high-quality, cost-effective healthcare. The challenge for a manager of human resources therefore is to recruit the best and keep them motivated. Scientific management will not work in modern oral healthcare delivery, even if it is a tradition. Practice owners and managers need to apply the theories of Maslow and Herzberg in order to maintain staff and practice quality and to remain competitive in the face of economic challenge.

# THE IMPORTANCE OF PLANNING

Planning is a key element in staff management. The planning group will have to make clear in the mission, goals, and objectives the value that the practice places on employees. If you are in a high-volume practice, where the emphasis is on production and not individualized service for each client, a high rate of staff turnover may be acceptable. If the practice is under extreme economic pressure and the highest priority objective is to control costs, with the alternative being to go out of business, you may have to accept high staff turnover as a consequence of cutting salaries and benefits. In any case, the first step is to decide what your mission, goals, and objectives are and then to plan accordingly. Don't begin at the end by cutting overhead expenses, resulting in staff turnover, and then realize that this is not in keeping with your plan. Consider several examples of practices in different situations.

## High Production

While not all practitioners, and probably not many students, would find a high-volume, production-oriented practice to their liking, there is no doubt that many such practices do exist. In low-income or underserved areas, such high-volume practices at least offer some access to oral healthcare. And while you may not find the thought of being a clinician in such a practice appealing, being a manager in a high-volume practice can be an exciting challenge. Whatever the case, it is useful for the manager to understand how to operate in such a setting. Chapters 8 and 9 will discuss managing finance and marketing in more detail. A high-volume practice requires careful financial management and aggressive marketing to be successful. Human resource management in such a setting requires considerable skill.

Goals and objectives that give priority to the maximization of profits and to the quantity of clients treated characterize a high-volume practice. Providing quality care may also be a goal, but it may have to assume a lower priority than profits and production, especially early in the practice life. The strategic plan must include strategies either for dealing with staff turnover or for providing adequate resources (training and equipment) and compensation (salaries and other benefits) for employees to enable the practice to keep the best on staff long term. As discussed previously, the best motivators will be more intangible, such as recognition of achievements, autonomy, opportunities for growth, and challenging and creative work.

In a high-volume, production-oriented practice, employees are under pressure to work as fast and as efficiently as possible. This pace increases the chances that employees, especially clinicians, may "burn out." Burnout describes a syndrome whereby employees grow tired, bored, and frustrated with their jobs, leading to lack of motivation, poor performance, decreased productivity, or any combination of these. You should anticipate and plan for or prevent burnout or turnover in order to meet your goals and objectives. Furthermore, the staff will be aware of the quantity of clients being treated and fees being collected and so may demand increased compensation.

How can the manager of the practice plan for these anticipated problems? If your strategic plan gives priority to profit making, you should keep overhead costs, especially salaries and benefits, to a minimum, as they comprise the bulk of the practice's operating expenses. If the salaries and benefits are low and the pressure to produce is high, you can probably anticipate a significant rate of staff turnover, along with its associated costs. You should analyze the finances of the practice to find the point at which handling staff turnover is cost effective. For example, if you find that the *total cost* of changing hygienists equals 12% of the expenses of the DHPC (see Chapter 2 for a discussion of the costs associated with staff changes), you would save quite a bit by keeping the existing staff and increasing the hygienists' compensation 5%. If, however, the *total cost* of changing hygienists equals 5% of the expenses of the DHPC and the hygienists are asking for a 10% increase in compensation, it will be cost effective to hire new hygienists.

If your analysis and strategic planning lead you to conclude that the goals and objectives of the practice will best be met by maintaining a stable staff, you will want to decrease the risk of burnout. There are steps that management can take to reduce employee burnout and keep the staff motivated. Increasing salaries is often not the best solution. Maslow's theory tells us that salary and job security are lower-order needs, and Herzberg's theory tells us that these are maintenance factors. Thus you should provide your employees with adequate salaries to meet their lower-level and maintenance needs for food, shelter, security, and a stable life, not necessarily the highest salaries in the area. Salaries that are competitive, in the low end to middle of the normal range, for your area and industry should be adequate to prevent job dissatisfaction. However, competitive salaries will not provide employee motivation or prevent burnout.

In a high-volume practice, where the risk of burnout and staff turnover is high, motivation is critical to maintaining a stable staff. Management must therefore address the higher-order needs and motivational factors of employees. This means publicly recognizing outstanding performance; offering responsibility, authority, and challenging work, advancement opportunities; and encouraging creativity. Some ways to achieve this include profit-sharing or bonus systems, a staff bulletin board or newsletter, opportunities for training, continuing education, and professional association involvement. Other rewards, such as gift certificates or dining out, may be effective if they are related to recognition of outstanding achievement. Listen to your employees. They are the best source of information about what will motivate them. While this approach to providing motivation and preventing burnout applies to all practices, it is especially critical in high-pressure situations.

This brings us back to planning. As you can see from the preceding discussion, keeping employees and motivating them costs the practice money. You must decide what your priorities are and, during the planning process, make the necessary trade-offs to achieve your objectives.

## Financial Crisis

Any practice may face a financial crisis. If your situational analysis is very good and you are very lucky, you may see the crisis coming in time to make changes to your strategic plan in advance. If not, you will have to rearrange your priorities in a hurry to stay in business. In either case, take time to consider your mission and goals and then modify your plan in a way that best suits your mission. If profits are your highest priority, ethics will prevent quality from suffering too much, but you will have to make compromises in a number of areas. If quality care is your highest priority, profits may have to suffer, but you will still have to find a way to keep the doors open without engaging in excessive borrowing.

If your practice is facing a financial crisis, you have three options: increase income, decrease expenses, or borrow. Your course of action will depend on the cause of the crisis. Borrowing might be the fastest solution, with the fewest short-term negative effects on the practice. You will have to eventually repay the money, so you must also consider the long-range consequences. Borrowing money is frequently quite difficult for small businesses, especially those with few fixed assets or little equity in their fixed assets. Increasing income quickly is usually hard in a service business, where development of a large client base takes time. If, however, you don't need to generate a lot of cash, and you have the resources, a quick, concentrated marketing effort may work.

Chances are you will have to reduce expenses and this means reducing operating costs. For a service business, where most of the operating costs go for human resources, staff reductions will probably be your only alternative. If you practice participative management, the entire staff may be involved in making these decisions. It would be a rare group that could actually come to consensus on layoffs. In the end, in any practice, owners and management will probably be responsible for the most painful or risky decisions. This is why the owners have invested in employing good managers.

Depending on the financial situation, it may be possible to keep staff reductions to a minimum by reducing compensation, either salaries or other benefits. Health insurance, for example, is a significant expense for most small businesses, but total loss of health insurance benefits can be devastating to an employee. Reduction of benefits, or increased employee contributions, is generally more acceptable than loss of insurance. Reduced compensation can be a winning approach for everyone involved. It is not beneficial, however, to keep on the staff employees who are disgruntled about reduced compensation. They can poison the emotional environment and this is the last thing you need in the midst of a financial crisis. It is better to lay off or fire employees who cannot or will not accept reductions in salary and/or benefits with a positive attitude.

Depending on your strategic plan, the best way to meet your goals in the face of financial crisis may be to reduce staff. If staff reduction is necessary, make logical decisions, not emotional ones. Base your choices on finding the most efficient way to follow your mission and make progress toward your goals. Keep the employees who are most critical to the survival of the business and who are the best at what they do. Let the rest go as amicably and quickly as possible. Remember that the crisis will put considerable strain on the employees that remain. You will have to plan to prevent burnout and allow for the associated costs.

The employees most critical to survival are the clinicians because they provide the services that generate the income. You must develop a plan that keeps income at the highest possible level and this means keeping as many clinicians working as you can. You probably will have no options other than to decrease support personnel or services. This will decrease the efficiency of the remaining clinicians, who will also have to complete the tasks of the missing support personnel. As in the situation where compensation was decreased, you should keep only the clinicians who can adjust to the necessary changes with a positive attitude and terminate, as soon as possible, the employment of those who can't adjust.

If you have a good working group, it is possible to pull through a financial crisis and its associated hardships with most of your best staff members in place and with minimal effect on moral. If you can involve the staff in making some of the difficult critical decisions, your chances of producing positive results may improve. However, it is one thing to ask your staff to pull together and make sacrifices in a crisis and quite another to fake or exaggerate a crisis in order to win concessions from employees. The best and brightest will catch on quickly and leave as soon as possible. In the end, such tactics can only make a difficult situation worse. It is best to be honest with your employees about the strategic plan from the beginning. You will then have a staff who knows what to expect, understands the big picture, and agrees with your practice philosophy.

## Small or Start-Up Practice

A small practice or start-up operation may have only one or two part-time employees. Unless the practice is buying out an established practice that can supply a constant stream of clients, the practice manager will face some combination of all the challenges discussed in the High Production and Financial Crisis sections. In the small or start-up practice, the pressures of the high-volume practice will be created because of the need to build the practice by bringing in new clients. Financial crises will occur when the flow of new clients into the practice is not sufficient to keep income at the necessary level. You will have to deal with these problems as discussed in the preceding sections.

If your practice has limited resources and an uncertain supply of clients, planning will be critical. Your strategic plan will have to include best- and worst-case projections and strategies to deal with each situation. Preparing coping strategies in advance will give you some advantage when a problem arises. You will spend less time on analysis and brainstorming and can move right into action mode to prevent the problem from becoming worse. Managing cash flow is usually the most difficult challenge in a small business, especially in a new one (see Chapter 3, Managing Cash Flow). Keeping the few staff members involved and informed will increase the likelihood of your having employees who can weather the storms of small business and still enjoy their jobs.

# COMPENSATION

There are many methods of compensation for various oral healthcare providers and staff members. Hygienists and dentists generate the income and so a large percentage of the operating expenses is their compensation (salary and benefits). Clinicians may be paid in a variety of ways including hourly, salary, commission, or some combination of these. Compensation methods for practice owners or partners may be more complicated, the details of which should be delineated in a contract. The following discussion pertains to employees of the practice.

The ADHA *Practices and Procedures Survey* (1988) reported data on methods of compensation for dental hygienists. They found that among hygienists working in dental offices, 32% were paid on an hourly basis, 37% were paid on a daily basis, 24% were paid a salary, 19% were paid commission, and 8% were paid a salary plus commission. Hygienists were more likely to be paid on an hourly basis if they worked in practices with large numbers of personnel.

Compensation arrangements for dentist-employees may differ from that of hygienists. Dental procedures generally produce more income for the practice, although profit margins for dental and dental hygiene services may be similar. Dentist-employees are more likely to ask for commission or salary plus commission. If you are unsure of your financial projections regarding new employee-dentists, limit your exposure. Negotiate the lowest possible compensation arrangement—you can always renegotiate and increase compensation after a few months. Increasing compensation is always easier than decreasing it. Don't get yourself into a situation where the dentist-employee is costing the practice more income than she is producing.

Often, other employees are paid by the hour for the exact numbers of hours worked, less any time off for breaks or meals. Hourly employees are nonexempt, and in some industries, nonexempt employees are paid extra for working more than full-time hours. Full-time varies from business to business, but is usually about 28 (the federal minimum) to 40 hours per week. Nonexempt employees may be paid time and half (the base pay plus 50%) or double time (200% of base pay) for overtime. They may also be paid higher rates for working evenings or weekends, although this is rarely the case for nonexempt dental hygienists.

For the practice, the advantage of having hourly, nonexempt employees who are not paid overtime is that you will save on wages. However, if you are located in an area with a highly competitive employment market, overtime pay might be a good incentive to retain or recruit remarkable employees. If you are having trouble convincing hygienists (or assistants) to work evening or Saturday hours, increased salary may be a good way to recognize their efforts on behalf of the practice.

Some practices charge a premium for evening or Saturday appointments. This practice helps to defray the costs involved for the practice, emphasizes, for clients, the value of these appointment times, and decreases the incidence of cancellations and missed appointments.

Employees on salary work a full work period for a specified salary, making them exempt. Exempt employees are not paid overtime and are expected to work as many hours as necessary to get the job done. One advantage of paying salaries is that payroll amounts for the exempt employees do not vary and so may simplify cash flow projections and bookkeeping procedures. In a practice with responsible employees, paying them on salary works well. The best employees to pay on salary are those who fulfill their obligations to complete work as necessary and those clinicians with marketing or public relations responsibilities outside their regular clinical duties. You'll save money on overtime, especially during busy periods. The negative impact will occur if you have many unfilled appointments or cancellations, because you will be obliged to pay the clinicians their full pay for the period, regardless of how much income they generate.

Commission is paid as a percentage of sales, either gross or net, depending on the arrangement. For example, a hygienist working on 40% commission who grossed $2800 in a week would receive $1120, leaving the practice $1680 in gross profit. In a very busy practice, commission payments could be considerable. Having dentists or hygienists work on commission alone gives them considerable motivation to build the practice, work efficiently, and keep their schedules full. For a start-up or slow practice, this can be important. It can also keep a busy practice moving well. Another advantage is that the practice does not have to pay for the clinicians' time if there are cancellations or unfilled appointments. Paying on commission only ensures that dentists and hygienists must always generate income greater than their compensation expenses.

Suppose a salaried hygienist earned $720 per week and generated $2800 with a full schedule. Assuming it cost the practice an additional 30% of her salary in payroll taxes and so on, the practice would spend a total of about $936 on her compensation that week. On the other hand, if only half of the schedule were filled, the hygienist would only generate $1400 that week. Considering compensation only, no other overhead expenses, the practice would net $464 for the week. With other overhead expenses factored in, it might actually cost the practice more to employ the hygienist that week than she produced in income. The practice would be obligated to pay the hygienist's salary regardless of production.

If, in the same practice, the hygienist were paid on commission only (40% of gross) and generated $2800 in revenue, it would cost the practice about $1456 ($1120 + 30%) in compensation, leaving the practice $1344 in profit. But if the hygienist only produced $1400 in one week, it would cost the practice only $728 ($560 + 30%) in compensation, leaving the practice $672, compared to $464 for the same case with a salaried hygienist. Similar projections could be made for a dentist's compensation.

Some hygienists and dentists are paid a combination of salary plus commission. In this way, they are guaranteed some base pay (usually much lower than what would be paid to someone on salary only) plus commission. The commission may be based on gross or net or may be effective only after some minimum level of production is achieved. This system can provide the advantages of salary and commission to both the clinicians and the practice.

A similar method of compensation involves bonus payments. Usually these systems operate so that employees are paid a percentage of profits. Often bonus systems go into effect only after profits exceed a specified level, so that the practice is not obligated to pay bonuses on falling production. This scheme is similar to profit sharing. As with commissions, bonus systems offer employees some direct incentives to work efficiently and increase production. Neither bonuses nor commissions, as described, offer any direct incentive to increase quality.

Although these methods of compensation have been discussed as they pertain to hygienists and dentists, they might be applied to any employee in the practice, although usually only hygienists and dentists work on commission. As mentioned in Chapter 3, there are tax implications involved in offering bonus or profit-sharing systems and the tax structure on commission payments differs from that on salary. Seek qualified financial advice in establishing these systems, for failure to comply with tax codes may result in significant tax liabilities for your business.

Although much of the discussion in this section focused on compensation, it is important to keep in mind the previous discussion of motivating factors. While employees need to earn enough to support themselves, money is not their main motivational issue. Motivating people involves respecting their professional opinions, giving them responsibility and authority for their work, and recognizing their contributions to the practice and the community. Remember that the employee working to fulfill higher-level needs for esteem and self-actualization will contribute the most to the practice.

# STAFF POSITIONS

Keep in mind that the best source of information about your employees is your employees. A book can only generalize. Human resource management decisions must depend mostly on input from your employees, not on information from any book or seminar. While management training can provide a strong background for dealing with people, there can be no substitute for knowing your practice, your employees, and your market.

## Managers

Hygienists and dentists have educational backgrounds in communications, human relations, education, and motivation, all valuable management skills. They understand the work of oral healthcare delivery. They understand, from first-hand experience, the importance of positive communication with clients. Compensation for managers may differ in amount and form from compensation for clinicians (dentists and hygienists).

First consider the sources of income and expenses in oral healthcare delivery. Clinicians generate the bulk of the income by providing services and should generate more income than expenses. The time they spend working is directly related to the amount of income generated, so the more clinicians work, the more income they generate (theoretically). Their time is directly billable. All other employees do not directly generate any income. The more they work, the more they are paid, without any direct proportional increase in income to the practice. They are paid out of operating expenses. This status is often referred to as being "on overhead."

The manager at start-up of many dental practices was the owner-dentist. The receptionist was the only person in the office doing any nonclinical work, and so the position of office manager evolved from the reception job, probably the lowest pay scale in the office. In some practices, the office manager evolved from an assistant who used some of her downtime to do purchasing and scheduling. Again, these were jobs usually low on the pay scale and contributed to the evolution of a tradition of low-paying management jobs in dental practice.

Hygienists and dentists may not evolve into office managers because almost all of their time is taken up by clinical responsibilities. Also, and especially in a new practice, a clinician can make the most valuable financial contribution to the business by treating clients since this generates income. Receptionists and assistants are already on overhead and receive lower pay than hygienists and dentists, and so it may be less painful financially to move them into office management, another overhead position. To move a hygienist, with a hygienist's salary, into management, and therefore onto overhead, can create a difficult financial situation. Not only does the practice lose the income the hygienist was bringing in, it has the added expense of paying a new staff member totally on overhead. Because dentists' compensation is usually significantly higher than hygienists', such a move for a dentist would be beyond the resources of most practices.

This common sequence of events, from lower-paying positions to pseudo-manager, may help to explain why dental practice managers are often at the low end of the pay scale and without specific management backgrounds. There is a flaw in this traditional logic. The best person for a management job is not necessarily the cheapest one you can find or the one with the most free time. The best person to manage any group, profit center, or dental practice is the one with the best skills, experience, and dedication to the business mission. This may be a dental hygienist, assistant, dentist, receptionist, or person from outside oral healthcare delivery. To receive adequate compensation, a dentist-manager would probably have to provide clinical services in addition. While it certainly makes sense to give receptionists or assistants expanded responsibilities, it does not automatically follow that any individual receptionist or assistant will be a good manager, just as it is not true that any hygienist or dentist will automatically be a good manager. With the right training and experience, however, many people from clinical backgrounds can become good managers.

A true manager is responsible for more than planning, organizing, controlling, and directing operations. The best practice managers are leaders who make things happen, who ensure that the business prospers and that the work environment is positive for employees and clients. An effective manager can make the difference between being barely profitable and being wildly successful. This is the value that a good manager brings to any practice.

The question to ask in choosing a practice manager is not "Who is cheapest?" but "Who can add the most value to this business?" This does not mean that you should pay more than the manager is worth. It means that compensation should be based on performance. If the practice manager can increase profits 300% and hiring the best only increases operating expenses 20%, you have made a wise investment. However, cash flow restraints may prevent you from bringing in a manager at a high pay scale. As already discussed, compensation can take forms other than straight salary. Commission, profit-sharing, and bonus systems reward performance but give the business the option of delaying cash expenditures until after payments are received. Sharing clinical and management duties reduces the financial impact, but part-time management is not always successful. This is one reason that many practices with only the dentist-owner as manager have so many problems.

For example, suppose the business owners decide that a dental hygienist is the person they want for practice manager. The cash-flow situation dictates that they must hire her at a salary level below that of the average clinical dental hygienist. By going with a bonus system, the practice has minimized its financial risk. If the manager successfully increases profits, she will increase her own compensation. If not, at least the business has not committed to paying her more than it can afford.

As the hygienist-manager increases profits, her compensation will increase through the bonus system. She will generate the cash flow to cover the increase in her own compensation and, additionally, will have financial incentives to do so. The potential exists that, with time, the hygienist-manager's total compensation will exceed that of a clinical dental hygienist.

In the preceding example, the practice owners were looking for increased profits and structured the manager's compensation to encourage this result. Another practice might have adequate profits but want a manager who can increase quality. In this case, the manager's compensation increases could be linked to quality measures. This scheme is a little riskier for the practice because it commits the business to increased expenses that may not be associated with increased income. A practice with strong profits and poor quality is in a good position to initialize a quality improvement plan. Making these choices will be part of the planning process.

## Dentists

Dentists may be associated with a dental practice in a number of ways, such as owner, partner, associate, employee (full-time or part-time), consultant, or manager. The positions and numbers of dentists employed by a practice will be a function of all the factors affecting the practice, including its mission, market, finances, and interests of the owners. Dentists who own all or part of a practice can be compensated in different ways, by taking the profits of the practice (if it is a sole proprietorship or simple partnership), or as contract employees (compensation arrangements defined by a contract) or employees-at-will (employees without contracts).

Whatever the relationship of a dentist to a dental practice (except sole owner), it is best to have a contract specifying the terms of the arrangement. The contract should be prepared only with the help of a qualified attorney experienced in dental practices. Check the references of the attorney or firm before working with them. The contract should cover all the issues, whether or not anyone believes there may be problems in the future.

Two areas of specific concern are noncompetition and nondisclosure clauses. Clients make a dental practice. If a dentist who has been part of your practice leaves, goes into competition with you, and takes many of your clients, your practice will have serious problems. A carefully drafted noncompetition clause can prevent most of these problems. Even if the dentist who leaves does compete with you, the noncompetition clause in the contract may give you legal rights to fair compensation. Nondisclosure clauses are less important for private practice, but vital for many types of businesses, especially those developing proprietary products. The purpose of the nondisclosure clause is to prevent an employee leaving your business from revealing any trade secrets or confidential information to competitors.

Other issues to cover in a contract with a dentist are those discussed in Chapter 2 and in this chapter pertaining to employment policies, such as compensation (salary, commission, bonus), leave, and other benefits (profit sharing, insurance, etc.). Failure to establish a firm, clear contract with any dentist associated with your dental practice can lead to serious trouble in the long run.

A DHPC that employs a dentist is a rarity, but liberal supervision requirements in some states might make such an arrangement feasible. Let's examine the pros and cons of having a DHPC employ a dentist. Dentists' salaries are generally higher than those of hygienists and assistants, so hiring a dentist, either as a contract employee or an employee-at-will, represents a substantial financial commitment for the DHPC.

One reason for the DHPC to contract with a dentist would be to provide supervision for hygienists to comply with legal restrictions. If a dentist in the DHPC spends all her time supervising hygienists and not doing any dentistry, she will not generate any income. If the dentist is earning a salary competitive with other dentists in the area, this will be prohibitively expensive. A more cost-effective arrangement would have the dentist practice dentistry, thereby generating income, and supervise hygienists. This would create a dental profit center and a dental practice. The most cost-effective arrangement would seem to be to operate the two profit centers separately, with each contracting for specific services from the other. This is a more traditional sort of practice and demonstrates why the traditional arrangement has proven to be popular and generally successful. You will, however, be able to find examples of successful nontraditional practices. A key to success in small business is to find an innovative solution to a problem. It will be up to the practice managers of the future to discover creative new practice modalities.

In the most common and traditional practice setting, the DHPC is part of a dental practice. The manager of the DHPC will not be responsible for the overall management of dentists but facilitating the interaction of supervising or consulting dentists within the DHPC. During the development of the strategic plan, the planning group will have to decide what specific sort of interaction is needed between the dentists and the DHPC. Much of this will depend on the philosophies of all the parties involved. The secret to achieving smooth, harmonious operations and consistent, comprehensive quality oral healthcare will depend upon finding a philosophy and plan that are enthusiastically supported by everyone involved.

Clients will be most "attached" to the healthcare providers, dental hygienists, and dentists. After all, the client has come seeking, and is paying for, the expertise of the clinicians. It is therefore important when making staffing decisions to strive to keep the providers in place. The practice manager will have to work with the hygienists and dentists to minimize turnover while being true to the mission and goals of the practice.

## Hygienists

A dental hygiene profit center provides dental hygiene services, so, by definition, a DHPC must include at least one hygienist; dental hygienists will be the principal clinicians in the DHPC. Statistically, the most likely setting for the DHPC will be in a dental practice (ADHA, 1988), so dentists will also function, for at least part of their time, within the DHPC. Dental assistants may also be involved in the DHPC, either peripherally or as dental hygiene assistants. Some type of office staff, for reception, billing, and filing, will also be necessary. As discussed in Chapter 6, even if these various staff members do not work solely within the DHPC, their input must still be considered as part of the overall operation of the DHPC. The manager must therefore be sensitive to management issues specific to these different roles.

The DHPC may employ any number of dental hygienists, depending on the strategic plan and resources. Dental hygienists, especially those with baccalaureate degrees, have a fairly broad general background and as such may fill roles other than clinician. The American Dental Hygienists' Association (1988) lists six roles for dental hygienists: manager, clinician, educator, researcher, change agent, and patient advocate. Depending on the DHPC practice setting, the hygienists may be filling a number of these roles. The work of dental hygiene clinicians is covered in detail in other dental hygiene texts; Part 3 will discuss dental hygienists in nonclinical management roles. There is little formal training available to fill the roles of change agent (a legislative activist) or patient advocate. These are roles that, by virtue of their educational backgrounds, hygienists may be prepared to assume, but much of the training is experiential. Depending on the practice setting of the DHPC, it may be advantageous to recruit hygienists with experience in one or some combination of the six roles.

## Assistants

A discussion of assistants in the DHPC is usually associated with a discussion of accelerated practice. The discussion of accelerated dental hygiene practice in Chapter 6 listed a variety of functions that assistants might perform in the practice. In an accelerated practice, the assistants would probably be performing all such functions that are legal in the practice location. In a more traditional type of practice, assistants might still perform some of these procedures, though they might not work full time in the DHPC. The role of assistants in your DHPC will depend on several factors, including your strategic plan, the resources available to the practice, and the experience and interests of the assistants themselves. The fact that hygienists have traditionally worked without assistants doesn't mean that such a collaboration cannot be enjoyable, cost effective, or productive. If assistants within your practice are not currently working in the DHPC but have some downtime or special interest, the staff may be able to create some new roles for assistants in the DHPC.

One role for assistants in the DHPC is often overlooked: business partner. Although business management may not be a regular part of an assistant's education, some assistants do come into the field with previous business experience or have been dental practice managers. Hygienists and assistants face similar challenges in practice and both may suffer from burnout. Such hygienists from traditional dental hygiene practice often explore independent contracting or other nontraditional business arrangements. Assistants are a group with similar interests and may find a challenge in partnership or management of a nontraditional DHPC.

Assistants in dental practice are essential. A dentist can work so much more efficiently with an assistant than without one that it is almost always cost effective to have a dental assistant. It is possible to arrange work loads so that the ratio of assistants to dentists does not have to be 1:1. One person could probably assist two or three dentists, if the proper equipment and support systems were in place and the assistant did not have general office duties as well. On the other hand, there can be many advantages to having assistant-to-dentist ratios greater than 1:1. If the practice is in a location where it can employ expanded-function assistants, this arrangement is usually cost effective. Expanded-function assistants can be trained for orthodontic or restorative procedures.

Whether you choose to employ expanded-function assistants will depend on your practice's mission, market, and resources. Because dentists are more highly paid than assistants, it is less costly to the practice to employ assistants to provide as many services as possible. In a very busy practice or an isolated one trying to serve an entire community, offering increased access to care is important for clients. If you are concerned, your practice can develop any necessary quality assurance mechanisms you feel are necessary.

While you want to keep assistants functioning at as high a level as possible, it is important to give them adequate and up-to-date training. Unless there are staff members in your practice with specific backgrounds in education, the assistants should be trained by those outside the practice specializing in dental assisting expanded functions. Furthermore, no employee should ever be asked to perform illegal duties. Dental assistants are not licensed, and in most states they are not required by law to be familiar with the dental or dental hygiene practice act. It is therefore the responsibility of management and licensed dentists and hygienists to be sure that their assistants are not practicing illegally. Furthermore, if any licensing board becomes aware of assistants operating illegally in your practice, action will be taken against the license of the *employer*.

Expanded duty or not, all assistants should participate regularly in continuing education and other training programs, as should all employees. Clients may become just as attached to the assistants as they are to the dentists and hygienists. Job turnover among assistants should be minimized, for marketing purposes and to decrease stress on the rest of the staff. Although assistants are not direct care providers, and are therefore working on overhead, you cannot keep the best if you are not meeting their needs and providing adequate motivating factors (as discussed in the first part of this chapter).

## Office Support Staff

The practice may assign employees to phone duties, appointment scheduling, billing, collections, filing, or related office duties. These functions may be assigned to one person or many. Because the office support staff, such as the receptionist or insurance claims processor, may be key contacts for clients, it is critical that they be well trained in their functions and in client interaction as well. The practice manager will be responsible for ensuring that the office support staff has adequate training in issues and procedures specific to that practice and specialty, if applicable.

Consider an example of a traditional dental practice, where the DHPC is an integral part of the dental practice and there are no hygiene assistants. Office support staff will still need specific training in working with the DHPC. The following discussion could also apply to a dental specialty practice or to another profit center within a general dental practice. Scheduling for hygiene clients will not be the same as scheduling for dental clients. A hygienist working alone will require more time to complete a procedure, such as ultrasonic scaling, than a dentist working with an assistant. Also, the unassisted hygienist, working out of one treatment room, will need more time between clients to clean and complete infection-control procedures. A dentist, working with an assistant out of two treatment rooms, can move between clients much more quickly. The person scheduling appointments needs to understand these subtle differences and the procedures for booking time appropriately.

Billing and insurance claim processing provide other examples. In a dental practice with a DHPC, it would be most cost effective to schedule periodontal initial therapy visits in the DHPC. This would mean multiple appointments with the hygienist for quadrant scaling, antimicrobial irrigation, and related procedures. Because this treatment is so complex and requires so many office visits, the person doing the billing and insurance processing will have to understand this aspect of dental hygiene treatment (and many others) to effectively process insurance claims and work out payment options with clients. Whether office staff are dedicated to the DHPC alone, or share time with other profit centers, the practice manager will have to be sure that all necessary staff members have up-to-date training and understand the operations of the practice in the areas for which they are responsible.

There is a danger that if office staff are not full time with one profit center, their work may be taken for granted by those most closely involved with profit center operations. Support functions are not often highly visible and it is easy for busy people to be unaware of their importance to smooth operations. Any employee whose work affects a profit center should be considered part of the profit center and should accordingly be involved in planning, training, and any other relevant meetings or activities for that profit center. All of the training activities for the various profit centers might be combined into one long session or might be divided by profit center, depending on the size of the staff.

Office support personnel often have the lowest pay scale because they do not contribute directly to production. However, support functions should be vital to production or they should be eliminated. If your practice is staffed correctly for support functions, you cannot afford to accept inferior work in this area any more than you can accept inferior clinical services. As is the case with other types of employees, the best person for the job is not the one willing to accept the lowest salary. The best person is the one most qualified and most likely to fit in with the mission, goals, and clients of the practice.

Employment issues, regardless of the type of employee involved, can be summarized by saying that you should hire the best. Train and keep training them. Provide adequate compensation and benefits. Find employees who are working to address their higher-order needs. Provide ample motivation. Respect your employees and train and motivate them to respect your clients. Keep all the employees involved in the decision-making process as much as possible. The payoffs will go far beyond good employee relations and smooth management. You will decrease expenses and increase income in the long run.

## Staff Meetings

Staff meetings are a necessity. Regardless of the size of your staff, some type of regular meetings is a must and the only possible way to implement most of the management techniques presented here. Time spent in meetings is not highly productive, so an experienced manager will limit the length of each meeting. Discussion will inevitably expand to fill the time allotted, but participants will be forced to stick to the issues and make decisions. This does not mean that you can't have open discussion, only that the meeting facilitator must keep the group on task. Generally, this means that the facilitator must limit her input or risk dominating the entire meeting.

One way to keep meetings on track is to prepare an agenda in advance. An agenda provides everyone involved with a chance to prepare for the discussion and may reduce premeeting anxiety about difficult issues. Additionally, it is helpful to save a copy of the agenda to document what was discussed, not just for your own records, but for compliance with outside regulations. OSHA and other safety and health regulations stipulate specific meeting and training requirements for the staff. The agenda and meeting records can serve as documentation for meeting these requirements and for staff involvement with such programs.

Involve all staff members in staff meetings, even part-time employees. It is the part-timers who must have this time to interact with the rest of the staff, because their work hours are limited. Encourage everyone in attendance to participate. Don't let some members dominate while others remain silent. This can lead to just about every imaginable kind of personnel management problem.

Never hold staff meetings while clients are in the office. First of all, if the entire staff is in the meeting, who is helping the clients? Second, you do not want your clients to be privy to the staff discussion. Hold the staff meetings in whatever area is large enough to hold everyone so that all participants can see one another. Do not have people seated theater style, with the facilitator at the front of the room. This is not conducive to open discussion. You may or may not choose to allow eating during the meetings. The decision will depend on the size of your facilities and staff. Try it both ways, if possible, and see what works best.

You can hold the staff meetings, on a regular basis, at any time convenient for the entire staff. Make it clear to part-timers when you hire them that they will be required to attend staff meetings. Staff meetings are a critical element in successful practice management and an important part of each employee's job. You must pay your nonexempt employees for time spent at staff meetings, even if the practice is providing refreshments. These meetings are a meaningful part of their work and participation should be mandatory. Don't make your nonexempt employees work for free. It is not good management and diminishes the importance of staff meetings.

Make whatever arrangements are necessary, but have regular, efficient meetings of the entire staff. Keep the tone positive, even if discussion of issues becomes heated. The meeting facilitator must be responsible for ensuring that staff meetings do not become gripe sessions. Two excellent references for meeting facilitators are Edward DeBono's *Six Thinking Hats* [1986] and *Six Action Shoes* [1992]. These two books outline simple procedures for directing group thinking in a positive manner, toward constructive action. You can schedule other meetings as needed, to discuss specific group, profit center, or individual issues. Most problems cannot be solved by ignoring them. Deal with issues directly, as they arise. The best opportunities for doing this may be informal (i.e., not during a regular staff meeting).

## Job Descriptions

A job description is just that—a description of the job. Usually the job description is one to two pages long and defines the responsibilities of the employee. The format of job descriptions may vary quite a bit from one practice to another, depending on the needs of the group.

Job descriptions can be used for a variety of purposes. As discussed in Chapter 2, the first use you might have for a job description is during the hiring process, to help clarify the requirements for the position being filled. You could also present the job description to employment candidates, so that they understand what is expected of them. It may also be a good idea to include a phrase such as "compliance with OSHA regulations is a condition of employment." This will give a clear message to employees of what is expected of them and clearly indicates that those who fail to comply may be disciplined or fired.

You can also use job descriptions during the planning process. As you develop strategies and action plans, referencing the job descriptions can simplify the planning. You will know, without having to consult with additional people, who is responsible for what. Additionally, during planning, you may be making decisions on expanding or reducing staff and you may need job descriptions to make informed decisions. Managers or employees may, during the course of implementing the plan, discover that job descriptions need to be modified. Going through the modification of the job description will help the parties involved focus their thinking about what needs to change. You can also refer to a job description when writing performance objectives. In a small business, all employees will probably be involved in planning and creating performance objectives, so you can do without the formal job descriptions.

You need to be aware that in many circles job descriptions are being eliminated on the grounds that they are too confining and inflexible. In an organization in which jobs are highly specialized, a pervasive "it's not in my job description" attitude can develop. In the end, it is the client who pays the price for this atmosphere. If all employees are focused totally on fulfilling just the responsibilities outlined in their own job descriptions, who is looking at the big picture? Who is looking out for the client? Any business that is not meeting the needs of its clients will eventually be out of business. The clients will go elsewhere and do business with someone who will meet their needs.

Everyone cares for clients. There will be times when something needs to be done that does not fall within anyone's job description or when the person who should be responsible isn't there. Who will take responsibility in unusual circumstances if everyone does only what's in her or his job description? In a group practice, with several dentists and dental hygienists, clients may get lost in the shuffle. The hygienist may think that a dentist in the practice is watching out for the clients' restorative needs and the dentist may be waiting for the hygienist to bring problems to her attention. Again, both the dentist and the hygienist are following their job descriptions. The hygienist is documenting the client's needs, and the dentist is providing restorations for clients in her schedule. Who is following the client to be sure that she is making necessary appointments?

Suppose a client has some minor complaint about the dentist and tells the hygienist? Who is responsible for dealing with the client's concern? It's not in the hygienist's job description that she should criticize the dentist's work. What will become of the client and her complaint? Eventually she will go elsewhere for treatment if her concerns are ignored. If everyone is responsible for being responsive to the client, regardless of individual duties, the client's concern would be addressed as quickly as possible by the first person she mentioned it to. The client would see that her interests come first in the practice.

Licensing and regulatory rules restrict the amount of overlap between job functions. Assistants, office support personnel, hygienists, and dentists cannot all legally provide the same services for clients. It is a responsibility of management and every licensed practitioner to ensure that every employee is working within the legal scope of practice. The practice act is something you need to review with all employees. All other job functions and employee responsibilities can be expounded in the mission statement, goals, objectives, and action plans. If the service attitude is an integral part of your practice philosophy (and it should be), this will be evident in every piece of your strategic plan. Especially in a small practice or profit center, job descriptions aren't necessary.

If you decide that the employees in your practice need job descriptions, keep the mission in mind. Be sure that each job description is broad enough to encompass the practice's mission and goals and remember that the job description may be viewed as an agreement between employer and employee. When you give the employee a job description, you are making a commitment that the person will not be asked to perform duties outside the job description, regardless of the situation. If you don't absolutely need job descriptions, work without them. You can probably accomplish all you want by involving all the employees in the planning process and in the creation of performance objectives.

## Employment Contracts

You may choose to use employment contracts in your practice. Typically, employment agreements (contracts) are used with dental hygienists, dentists, and, occasionally, assistants. You may, of course, use employment agreements with any employee you choose. There are advantages and disadvantages to doing so. Whether the advantages outweigh the disadvantages depends on your particular situation.

One of the advantages is that the manager of the practice, the employee, and the practice owners will have a clear, written account of their agreement. This may help improve communications among these parties and it may help prevent misunderstandings. An employment agreement does not, however, guarantee good communications or total understanding. All statements, written and verbal, are subject to the interpretation of the individuals reading or hearing them. Written statements do provide an advantage in that when questions arise as to the exact nature of the agreement, you can refer to the written record and do not have to rely on anyone's memory of what was said.

If you have a contract with an employee who quits suddenly, you will have some legal basis for action if the manner in which the employee quits violates the terms of the employment agreement. For example, if your contract dental hygienist quits at 8:00 A.M. on Monday morning, leaving you with a full schedule of clients and no one to treat them, the practice will suffer a financial loss. If the employment agreement requires a 10-day written notice to cancel the contract, you may be able to recover some compensation from the hygienist. For example, you may demand that she compensate the practice for the loss of income from canceling clients for 10 days. You may include a demand for additional damages for loss of goodwill from clients disgruntled about last-minute cancellations.

This type of demand will most likely involve the practice in some legal action. The court may or may not rule in your favor, and meanwhile, the practice will have incurred a significant legal bill. You will have to determine whether legal action will cost you more than your loss of income. Generally, it will probably be cheaper just to let the employee leave. The exception may be the case where the hygienist leaves your practice and moves to one close by, taking many of your clients with her.

As discussed under dentists' contracts, contracts that include noncompetition agreements may offer a significant advantage to the practice. A noncompetition agreement is an arrangement that stipulates that the employee will not compete with the employer under specific conditions. In the case of a dental practice, competition usually takes the form of luring clients away. The noncompetition agreement must be definite about the exact terms of noncompetition. It should state a time period and geographic location that applies. For example, a noncompetition agreement in which the employee agreed never to compete with the employer would probably not stand up in court. On the other hand, a noncompetition agreement that stipulated that the employee could not practice dental hygiene at any location within five miles of the employer's practice for three years would have a better chance of being deemed valid in court. You may, in some cases, be able to win a case of this type without having a written contract and/or a noncompetition agreement, but it will be more difficult. Having the noncompetition agreement is no guarantee of successful suit, however.

There may be disadvantages to using an employment agreement. When you sign an employment agreement with your employee, that employee becomes a contract employee. As discussed in Chapter 2, employees-at-will (those working without contract) can be dismissed at any time and you are not required to give any reason. Dismissing or changing the terms of employment of a contract employee is entirely different, for you and the employee are bound by the terms of the employment contract. There are unusual circumstances when this may create a problem for the practice. For example, you would want to fire immediately a contract employee for stealing drugs from the office, but would be prohibited unless there is some language to this effect in the employment agreement.

Don't be put off by the presentation of an employment agreement during the interview process. Take this as a sign of the candidate's business experience and serious interest in your practice. Writing employment agreements is not a task for the beginner. *You should have advice from an attorney experienced in preparing employment contracts for dental practices.* Do not write your own contracts or sign one written by an employee without legal advice. Of course, a legal opinion is no guarantee of successful litigation.

In your employment negotiations, remember that you must find a win/win solution. You want each person you hire to be with you as long as possible and to be dedicated to your practice. If you begin the employer–employee relationship with one party feeling that she has lost the employment contract negotiations, you will not be off to a good start toward building a strong association.

# THE POLICY MANUAL

The terms *policy* and *procedure* are used interchangeably in this chapter, as they were in Chapter 2. This may not be the case in all workplaces, so be sure that you are using the term correctly in your business setting.

Chapter 2 outlined the sections of a general-purpose policy manual. The following discussion will refine the general-purpose manual for use in private practice. You may also want to review the section on risk management in Chapter 2. Risk management procedures will apply in all practice settings. If the practice is part of a large business, remember that small-business exemptions, commonly applicable in private practices, will not apply. Separate profit centers may not need their own policy manuals. For example, if the DHPC is operated as an integral part of another practice, the policy manual for the practice will cover the operation of the DHPC as well.

The following descriptions list the sections the practice policy manual might include.

## Rules and Regulations

This section can contain general guidelines for the work environment. It may also include a list of serious offenses for which there are immediate consequences. A code of ethics might be in this section or listed separately. You may use a professional code or your practice may have its own.

If the practice has rules about wearing uniforms or professional appearance, they should be included. If there are rules or standards, they must be applied consistently. If the practice is fairly relaxed about these requirements, however, it is not necessary to have written policy on the matter.

## Occupational Safety and Health

Occupational Safety and Health Administration (OSHA) standards applicable to oral healthcare delivery are extensive. For a copy of the current OSHA standards, contact the U.S. Department of Labor and ask for "Controlling Occupational Exposure to Bloodborne Pathogens in Dentistry," U.S. Dept. of Labor, OSHA 3129, 1992, OSH Act of 1970, OSHA's standard for *Occupational Exposure to Bloodborne Pathogens*, December 6, 1991, Title 29 Code of Federal Regulations 1910.1030. There are also state safety and health standards that apply. Because these standards are extensive and quite specific and often include requirements related to documentation, it is best to maintain a separate OSHA manual and records. The practice must be in compliance with OSHA standards. The role of the practice manager will be to ensure that the practice and its employees are in compliance with all of the applicable state and federal requirements.

Because exposure-control procedures and documentation are extensive, you may choose to assign responsibility for overseeing this area to one person. This person need not be the practice manager, but another staff member with interest or expertise in exposure control. Whoever is responsible must have ongoing training in state-of-the-art procedures and authority to take action.

## Worker's Compensation

Employees who suffer a job-related injury may be eligible for benefits under worker's compensation, so including information about worker's comp in the policy manual is helpful. Because exposure to blood-borne pathogens and hazardous dental materials can cause serious work-related injuries, management needs to minimize these risks. Exposure control is part of the OSHA regulations, so these rules will probably be included with the OSHA manual, rather than in the policy manual.

A common job-related injury in dentistry and dental hygiene is carpal tunnel syndrome (CTS). CTS is a condition that occurs when the nerves of the hands are compressed as they pass through the carpal tunnel in the wrist (Gerwatowski, McFall, & Stach, 1992), often as a result of repetitive, flexing wrist motions. The symptoms of CTS may include pain, tingling, reduced sensation, numbness, weakness, and clumsiness of the hands. Those affected may be unable to perform job functions. If the employee can prove that the condition was caused by work, the employee may receive worker's compensation benefits. The benefit period may vary considerably from state to state and from case to case.

As mentioned in Chapter 2, the employer's contributions to worker's compensation are largely based on the number of claims filed by employees. Because these contributions can become very high, it is in the best interest of the employer to prevent work-related injuries from an economic as well as an ethical standpoint. The money invested to keep the workplace safe will probably pay for itself over time. In the case of CTS, there are many strategies to use to avoid its development (Gerwatowski, McFall, & Stach, 1992). The practice manager can encourage employees to attend relevant continuing education courses and can provide equipment designed to minimize wrist stress.

## Attendance and Punctuality

Attendance and punctuality can be critical performance issues in private practice. If the client schedule is carefully managed to be tight and efficient, late or absent employees can bring the entire system to a crashing halt. It is therefore advisable to have clearly defined policy on attendance and punctuality, with strict consequences for infractions. An employee whose work is outstanding but who is habitually late or missing will cause so many problems that the issue will have to be addressed and resolved promptly.

The policy manual should specify the correct procedure to call in sick. People often don't know they will be out sick until early morning, so it may be necessary for all employees to have the home phone number(s) of the person(s) they are to contact, although it may not be necessary to include phone numbers in the policy manual. You may want to consider having a phone list for the practice.

## Payroll

Specify what the paydays are. Explain payroll deductions for social security taxes, unemployment insurance, worker's compensation insurance, and federal and state income taxes. This section might also state the procedures to follow for payroll or tax questions, necessary changes, or disputes.

There may be payroll deductions for health insurance, life or disability insurance, or contributions to retirement plans. These benefits should be explained in detail in other areas of the policy manual, but it is a good idea to mention any applicable deductions in the payroll section so that employees can interpret their payroll checks by referring to this one place.

## Hours of Work

This section might list regular office hours. If you have part-time employees with varying schedules, and everyone's work hours are not the same, you may want to eliminate this section in the policy manual to avoid confusion. Just be sure that each employee does know when to come to work.

## Benefits

The practice can choose to offer from among a myriad of benefits: health, disability, malpractice, or life insurance; profit-sharing, pension, or retirement plans; reimbursement of continuing education fees; free parking; or uniform allowance. There are many others, depending on employee interest and practice resources. The policy manual should explain each program in detail, stating who is eligible, how benefits are administered, and the procedures for questions or problem resolution.

Private dental practices have traditionally been very stingy in offering employee benefits. This may be due to many factors, including a lack of specific management training or experience among practice owners. Oral healthcare delivery is a labor-intensive business, where the cost of goods sold and supplies are a much smaller percentage of total operating expenses than salaries and benefits. When looking for ways to increase the profit margin, the most obvious method is to reduce operating expenses by reducing or eliminating benefits because reducing the number of employees can be difficult in a labor-intensive business. The untrained or inexperienced may choose the most obvious solution without considering the hidden costs.

Poor benefits or inadequate compensation may lead to high rates of employee turnover. As discussed in Chapter 2, the costs involved in turnover can be high and may include the cost of recruiting, hiring, unemployment claims, training, lost clients, decreased market share, and bad public relations within the community, to name a few. Designing a cost-effective benefit package for your practice will depend on the goals and objectives of the practice and upon the value that management and employees place on employee benefits. Whatever the case, it is important that the policies be applied uniformly and consistently.

   Lack of benefits is often cited as a reason for dissatisfaction with employment among dental hygienists and dental assistants. Management has the authority and the responsibility to correct past mistakes and to apply modern management principles to oral healthcare delivery. This can improve the quality of employees attracted to the field and, by implication, the quality of care delivered.

## Overtime or Compensation Time

All employees should know whether they are exempt or nonexempt and eligible for overtime or comp time. Although overtime payment is common in many industries and comp time is used in some, traditional dental practices have not historically offered these benefits.

   If the practice is located within a large institution, such as a hospital, it is possible that some employment practices within the practice may be affected by union regulations. Union policies and procedures will probably be contained in a separate section or manual.

## Holiday Schedule

This section should contain a list of holidays for which employees will be paid. The policy might also delineate who is eligible for holiday pay. Typically, employees on unpaid leave do not receive holiday pay, but employees on paid leave do. Part-time employees may not be eligible for holiday pay, or the policy may be to pay them if the holiday falls on one of their regularly scheduled workdays. Holiday pay is often an issue in private dental practice. Delineating a policy and applying it consistently can prevent misunderstandings.

## Leave

This section of the policy manual should state the definitions of the types of leave recognized in the practice, how it is accrued, how it can be used, and how and when to get approval for taking it.

   You may also want to consider a system of wellness pay. Wellness pay is awarded to those employees who do not use any of their sick leave during a specified period. If you are paying some employees for time out sick, they are receiving a benefit that well employees are not. In essence, you are providing an incentive to be ill and miss work. A more positive approach is to offer an incentive for *not* missing work—wellness pay. Wellness pay is usually awarded in an amount equal to the standard amount of sick leave. For example, if, in your practice, employees can accrue 10 days of sick leave per year, the wellness pay award would be equal to 10 days' salary. Any employee who doesn't miss a day of work all year has made a considerable effort on behalf of the practice and deserves to be recognized and rewarded. Ten days' salary may seem like a significant amount of money, but consider the alternative. If the employee had missed 10 days of work, or even 2 or 3, how would this have affected the operating costs of the practice? You may find that a wellness pay program is cost effective.

## Technology

You should have policies on managing technology. Technology commonly used may include computers, audiovisual equipment, microscopes, x-ray equipment and processors, and an array of other clinical tools (lasers, ultrasonic scalers, electronic probes, etc.). This equipment, as well as all the other commonly used dental equipment, represents a significant capital investment for the practice owners, so following care and maintenance procedures is critical. Management is responsible for ensuring that all employees are properly trained on the use and care of all equipment they use.

Careful documentation of these procedures in the policy manual is helpful, but training is also required. The use and care of specific pieces of equipment or systems will probably be covered in users' manuals. Initial training is usually not sufficient. To make the workplace safer and reduce expenditures for equipment, keep all employees up to date by having periodic review. If there is some penalty for misuse of or damage to equipment, include all the details in the procedure manual. Be sure to apply penalties consistently.

The preceding discussion has given you some ideas of sections to include in a policy and procedure manual. The manual may need to be expanded or condensed, based on the needs of your particular business. Although all practices must have an OSHA manual, many small businesses can function without a policy manual. If the practice has only a few employees, all the appropriate policy and procedure information can be included in the job descriptions for each employee or discussed at staff meetings. This can be an advantage for management because it leaves you more flexible and unbound by written policies. Flexibility is an advantage in small business and can result in a friendly, casual work atmosphere. The disadvantage in not having written policies is that this may make it difficult to be consistent. Inconsistency can cause problems with employee morale and may pose some legal risks as well.

### *Summary*

Compensation is important, but while employees need to earn enough to support themselves, money is not the main motivational issue. Motivating people involves respecting their professional opinions, giving them responsibility and authority for their work, and recognizing their contributions to the practice and the community. Remember, the employee working to fulfill higher-level needs for esteem and self-actualization will contribute the most to the practice.

You should hire the best and then train and keep training them. Provide adequate compensation and benefits and find employees who are working to address their higher-order needs. Provide ample motivation. Respect your employees and train and motivate them to respect your clients. Keep all the employees involved in the decision-making process as much as possible. The payoffs will go far beyond good employee relations and smooth management. You will decrease expenses and increase income in the long run.

Your practice may need a policy/procedure manual. The policy manual can contain details of policies and procedures related to job functions and managing human resources. A small organization or one that is flat may function well without a policy manual, as long as procedures are fair and applied consistently. In an organization with good communications, operations may be more flexible and responsive in the absence of a written manual.

Oral healthcare delivery is a people-oriented business. The success of the practice will depend on its ability to be totally responsive to its clients and on the dedication of its employees.

## Review Questions

1. Compare and contrast Maslow's and Herzberg's theories of motivation.

2. Describe a situation in which your job performance or the job performance of someone you manage was adversely affected by a change in status that caused you/your employee to focus on filling one of Maslow's three lower-order needs.

3. Referring to Herzberg's theory, give an example of a situation in which a missing maintenance factor affected your performance or the performance of someone you know.

4. You are the manager of an accelerated practice. How will you meet your production goals without applying scientific management?

5. You are the manager in charge of starting a DHPC in a hospital dental clinic. What factors will you need to consider as you begin planning?

6. You are the manager of an established dental practice. Due to layoffs at a nearby factory, your business has decreased significantly. How will you alter your plan to cope with this setback?

7. Describe the type of compensation you would prefer to receive, and explain your reasons.

8. In the review questions for Chapter 2, you were asked to write a job description for a position that you have held. Was it helpful to you to have the job description? Would it have been helpful for your employer to use job descriptions? Why or why not?

9. When you are a practice manager, will you have your employees use job descriptions? Why or why not?

10. Discuss the impact of OSHA regulations on managing oral healthcare delivery.

11. Discuss ways in which OSHA regulations have impacted procedures in your office or school.

12. Describe how you, as manager of a practice, can motivate your employees to carefully follow all infection control procedures.

13. List at least six topics to include in a practice procedure manual and state your justification for including them.

14. The following review questions were used in Chapter 2. Now that you understand more, would you answer these questions differently? Why or why not?

    a. If you are currently employed, look at the policy or procedure manual at your office. If not, obtain one for your school or volunteer organization. Are any of the policies out of date? If so, why? Are new policies needed? In what areas?

    b. Write a new policy for one of the areas identified in part (a).

## SUGGESTED READING

American Dental Hygienists' Association. (1992). *Employment reference guide.* Chicago: ADHA.

Bassett, L. C., & Metzger, N. (1986). *Achieving excellence.* Rockville: Aspen Publications.

Campbell, P. R. (1989). Managerial role development of the dental hygienists in initial client interactions. *Journal of Dental Hygiene,* 63(7), 342–346.

Domer, L. R., Snyder, T. L., & Heid, D. W. (1980). *Dental practice management.* St. Louis: C.V. Mosby.

Liebler, J. G., Levine, R. E., & Rothman, J. (1992). *Management principles for health professionals.* Rockville: Aspen Publications.

Loiacono, C. (1989). Manager's guide to reducing dental hygiene turnover. *Journal of Dental Hygiene,* 63(7), 328–334.

McConnell, C. R. (1992). *The effective health care supervisor.* Rockville: Aspen Publications.

Merrill, H. F., ed. (1970). *Classics in management.* New York: American Management Association.

Weisbord, M. R. (1987). *Productive workplaces.* San Francisco: Jossey-Bass.

Woodall, I., & Bentley, J. M. (1983). *Legal, ethical and management aspects of the dental care system* (2nd ed.). St. Louis: C.V. Mosby.

## REFERENCES

American Dental Hygienists' Association. (1988). *Practices and procedures survey.* Chicago: ADHA.

DeBono, E. *Six thinking hats.* (1986). New York: Little, Brown Co.

DeBono, E. *Six action shoes.* (1992). New York: Harper Business Press.

Donnelly, J. H., Gibson, J. L. & Ivancevich, J. M. (1984). *Fundamentals of management.* Plano: Business Publications, pp. 310–320.

Gerwatowski, L. J., McFall, D. B., & Stach, D. J. (1992). Carpal tunnel syndrome: Risk factors and preventive strategies for the dental hygienist. *Journal of Dental Hygiene,* 66(2), 89–94.

Herzberg, F. (1971). *Work and the nature of man.* New York: World Publishing Co.

Maslow, H. (1970). *Motivation and personality* (2nd ed.). New York: Harper and Row.

Peters, T. (1987). *Thriving on chaos.* New York: Harper Perennial, pp. 80–81.

# CHAPTER 8

# Financial Management of Oral Healthcare Delivery

## Objectives

After reading this chapter and completing the review questions, the reader should be able to:

- Describe two methods of tracking productivity in the dental hygiene profit center.
- Describe two methods of tracking productivity in a dental profit center.
- Discuss the advantages and disadvantages of using detailed fee schedules.
- Define the payment cycle.
- Discuss three factors that influence the length of the payment cycle.
- Discuss three ways to reduce the length of the payment cycle.
- State one reason for achieving timely fee collections.
- Describe six possible expenses for dental hygiene or dental practice.
- Define profit.

Finance of oral healthcare delivery can be considered in two broad categories: income and expenses. Most income is produced by providing services. Some additional income may be generated by the sale of goods (such as home care devices or fluorides) or by other investments, but production is the main source of income for dental or dental hygiene practice.

A practice will have a variety of expenses, depending on the practice setting and business arrangements, including payroll, debt payments, rent, supplies, and equipment. Most dental and dental hygiene practices are operated for profit. Practices located in not-for-profit settings, such as public health clinics, are generally expected to keep expenses under control. Depending on funding sources, some may be expected to break even (the expenses equal the profits). Whatever the case, managers are expected to control finances consistent with the mission of the practice setting. When you subtract the expenses from the income, what remains is profit.

# INCOME

## Understanding Production

Oral healthcare delivery does not involve the creation of products. Most production revenues are generated by services provided. Services provided in the dental and dental hygiene profit centers will differ. Within a dental practice, services might be divided into several different profit centers, for example, crown and bridge, surgery, and general restorative. Productivity can be measured in different ways, depending on the mission and goals of the practice. It is important to have some production measurement system in place, regardless of the measurement method(s) used, in order to track and analyze activities.

One method of tracking production is to report fees collected. The effectiveness of the collections process has a significant impact on differences between fees billed and fees collected. Tracking fees collected gives a realistic estimate of practice or profit center income and, as a production measure, takes into account the business functions of the practice beyond clinical activities. The efficiency of billing, collections, and insurance claims processing depends on office support personnel. The method you choose to use depends on what you are trying to measure. If you are concerned only with the production of providers, monitoring fees collected will give you a biased result.

Production can be monitored by tracking fees billed. While this method is quick and simple, its usefulness is limited, for there can be a significant difference between what is billed and what is collected. Collection can be influenced by many factors, including the payment cycle, insurance claim processing, and credit card fees. All these factors affect when the cash actually goes into the practice account. The one advantage of tracking fees billed is that it gives a more accurate record of provider activity than does fees collected.

Production can be tracked by reporting services provided. This method yields the most information regarding the activities of providers and would correlate with the fees billed data, but it involves the most extensive record keeping. If the practice is already computerized, it should be fairly simple to record/report services provided.

Some profit centers can use client visits as a measure of production. If every client receives the same services and is charged the same fee, this can be an accurate measure of production. As mentioned earlier, in some settings, seeing as many patients as possible may indeed be a goal. For example, in a fluoride rinse program, each client would be receiving the same service and an objective might be to produce as many client visits as possible each day. Some preferred provider organizations are essentially only concerned with the number of patients treated. In these cases, the number of client visits would be the production measure to use.

In a traditional private practice setting, where there can be quite a bit of variation in fees and treatment from one client to another, monitoring the number of client visits would not give enough detail about operations to be a meaningful measure of productivity.

Productivity and profitability can vary from one profit center to another simply because different types of services are being provided. For this reason, it is often helpful to divide one practice into several different profit centers so that management can accurately track productivity and profitability in each area. With all possible profit centers combined, in contrast, it is difficult to identify poor performers or recognize outstanding achievement.

## PRODUCTION IN THE DENTAL HYGIENE PROFIT CENTER

The DHPC produces dental hygiene services. Two of the most commonly used production measures are fees and client visits, within which categories are found a variety of methods. Choose a method that suits the mission of your DHPC.

For example, a DHPC in a county public health department would not track production by reporting fees billed. Because most of its services are probably provided for free or for a minimal charge, the fees billed would have little relationship to the amount of service provided. Client visits or services provided would be better measures of production. Many public health programs are also operating under constraints to produce some measurable health benefit, such as a reduced incidence of caries. The production objectives in a public health setting might thus be related to measurement of treatment or program outcomes. On the other hand, the manager of a DHPC in a private dental practice might be very concerned about fees billed. This measurement is easy to generate on a daily basis. Just sum up the billing for the DHPC.

Regardless of the measurement method used, the DHPC must have some record of production and it should be a measure that is easy to record as part of daily operations. The DHPC should also have some regular system for monitoring quality, lest it become too production oriented.

## PRODUCTION IN THE DENTAL PROFIT CENTER

As mentioned earlier, dental services might be considered as several profit centers, depending on the type of practice involved. A specialty practice, such as endodontics, might not need this degree of specificity, but a general practice probably will. In a general practice, for example, some procedures, such as crown and bridge, are more time consuming and more profitable than others. Crown and bridge work uses up a lot of provider time, but it also has a greater profit margin than general restorative (fillings). If these services are considered as two separate profit centers, it will be possible to analyze internal financial reports more accurately. For example, a provider who spends as much time on a class 2 amalgam as on a crown preparation will have low productivity. If general restorative and crown and bridge are reported as separate profit centers, the weak point will be easier to identify.

Additionally, some profit centers may use more resources than others. For example, more working capital might be used in the crown and bridge profit center to cover lab costs. The crown and bridge profit center might also use more assistants' time. Reporting profit center operations separately enables management to see that resources are being allocated and used efficiently. The usefulness of such reports will depend on choosing the right production measurement method.

## Fees

Fee schedules, production, and production measurement are closely related. Selecting the methods to use for a particular practice will depend on the mission and goals of the practice. In some cases, different methods should be used for different profit centers within one practice setting, but it is generally best to use the same method for each profit center to avoid excessive record keeping.

### FEE SCHEDULE FOR THE DENTAL HYGIENE PROFIT CENTER

How should the fee schedule for the DHPC be structured? One commonly used method is to charge a cluster fee for dental hygiene visits. For example, there is one cluster fee for "adult recall" that incorporates all the charges for the most frequent set of services provided at an adult maintenance visit such as examination, oral hygiene instructions, scaling, subgingival irrigation, polishing, and fluoride treatment. There is a similar (usually lower) cluster fee for child maintenance visits.

There are both production and marketing disadvantages to this system. For example, every adult client may not get a fluoride treatment. Some adults may need two hours of scaling and root planing, and others may only need 30 minutes. There can be a great deal of variation in the number and scope of services provided for each client. Using cluster fees promotes the idea of providing each person exactly the same type of service, regardless of the client's oral health needs. If the DHPC uses cluster fees, it will be overcharging some patients and undercharging others and in the end may not even out to the advantage of the DHPC.

The marketing disadvantage in using cluster fees is that clients may tend to overlook the extent of service provided in the DHPC. If they see a cluster fee, they may think that everyone gets the same treatment and that all recall visits are the same—teeth cleaning. If all their appointments last 45 minutes, they may not see that their home care makes any difference. Even if the dental hygienist tells them about the efficacy of their home care practices, fee differences may make a more lasting impact.

In a fee-for-service DHPC, a better method of fee scheduling is to view each client visit as a composite of services provided and designate a fee for each service. For example, there would be a charge for scaling, a charge for polishing, a charge for oral hygiene instructions, and so forth. For many patients, the total charges for a maintenance visit might be the same as the cluster fee. However, the client who requires two hours of root planing would be charged (usually per quadrant) considerably more than the client who requires only light supragingival scaling, and the client who requires generalized, light subgingival scaling would fall somewhere in the middle.

There are several advantages to using a detailed fee schedule. It is fair to clients. They are charged for the care they receive, not some amount normalized for the entire population. The fee schedule becomes a more accurate representation of the production of the DHPC. Patients are given financial incentive to practice good home care (shorter appointments, less expense). Practitioners working on commission or bonus are given an incentive to maximize their scheduling efficiency.

Using a detailed fee schedule also makes it simpler to assign charges to the correct profit center. For example, if a dentist examines a dental hygiene client, that exam fee should be credited to the dental profit center. Other examples are services that require the use of specialized capital equipment, such as subgingival irrigation. If the DHPC uses a detailed fee schedule, you can easily go back through the financial records (especially if they are computerized) and record exactly how many times the irrigation equipment was used. This can help in creating accurate projections of the need for equipment maintenance or replacement. It can also help to identify underused capital equipment. You will have this information in the client charts, but chart audits can be time consuming and therefore costly. Of course, services provided can be recorded elsewhere, but keeping them all on one record makes the process more efficient.

Soft tissue management programs typically rely on detailed fee schedules and may include separate fees for root planing, irrigation, antimicrobial treatment, microscopic examination, and oral hygiene instructions. The fee schedule helps the clients realize all the services they have received and appreciate the extra care they are given. Another way you can use a detailed fee schedule is to accommodate variations in the length and spacing of appointments. Clients with good home care usually need short appointments and clients with poor home care need longer (or multiple) appointments. A client on a three-month maintenance schedule may require shorter appointments than a similar case on a 6- to 9-month schedule. Fees can be based on the case difficulty (and, by implication, the length of the appointment).

When working with a detailed fee schedule, it is important that practitioners and insurance claims processors understand each other's functions. Practitioners need to know how insurance companies pay for various treatments so that they can develop a treatment plan that the client can afford. Those responsible for completing the insurance claims need to understand the various treatment procedures so that they can file the claims correctly and optimize the benefits the clients receive.

The advantages of detailed fee schedules are applicable mostly to fee-for-service DHPCs. DHPCs in which a majority of patients belong to health maintenance organizations (HMOs) or preferred provider organizations (PPOs) might not find the detailed schedule as useful. Many HMOs and PPOs pay a flat fee for each maintenance visit, regardless of the number or scope of services provided. From a quality standpoint, you might also note that this manner of payment promotes the practice of treating each client as identical and completing each case as quickly as possible, regardless of the client's health needs.

## FEE SCHEDULE FOR THE DENTAL PROFIT CENTER
Fee schedules for dental services have traditionally been more detailed than fee schedules for dental hygiene services, partly because of the wider range of services dentists might perform, especially in a general practice. The advantages of using a detailed fee schedule for dental practice are similar to those for hygiene prac-

tice—an emphasis on individualized care, more detail provided for clients, equity in billing clients, possible production incentives for practitioners, and more detail for internal reports.

Because of the greater profit margin in most dental services, there may be some advantage in reducing detail in the fee schedule. Some dental services, such as root canals, crowns, bridges, and removable prosthetics, require multiple visits. Some procedures involve the services of outside dental laboratories, or specialized equipment, such as lasers. For all of these procedures, clients are billed for the dentist's time, for multiple visits, outside labor, supplies, and special equipment. The fees for these services, usually substantial, are usually cluster fees and include the charges for all the steps, supplies, and equipment required. Depending on the market, clients may enjoy paying one fee for a complex service, rather than being charged each time they walk in the door. Some clients or market segments may prefer to see a detailed breakdown of all the charges for complex procedures, so that they feel they are getting their money's worth. Some insurance carriers also require this kind of detail. How a practice chooses to structure and present the fee schedule then is mostly a marketing decision. The fees may have to be presented differently to different micro markets, even though the total of the detailed charges for a complex procedure is equal to the cluster fee.

## CASE FEES

Patients with complex oral health needs may require extensive treatment. These patients need a specific case presentation in which they discuss and choose their comprehensive treatment plan (see Chapter 10). In these cases, there may be a case fee for the entire course of treatment. In a general dental practice, the case fee may include the charges for several different profit centers, including dental hygiene. In a specialty practice, such as orthodontics, the case fee may include the charges for several years' worth of treatment. Again, the degree of detail to include in the fee depends on the market, client requirements, and insurance carrier specifications.

## DISCOUNTED FEES

In most for-profit practices, sometimes it is necessary to discount fees. Discounting fees may have a significant impact on income, so it is advisable to include the discount schedule in the strategic plan. Fees may be discounted for many reasons, including clients' inability to pay, insurance requirements, and traditional discounts for family, friends, employees, and health professionals.

Almost all healthcare practices get requests for free or discounted service for the indigent and uninsured. This is especially true for oral healthcare because of the large percentage of clients who do not have dental insurance, even if they do have health insurance. During the planning process, you must decide how to handle requests for care from the indigent and uninsured, consistent with the practice philosophy, mission, and goals. The financial impact of providing free or deeply discounted treatment depends on a number of factors, including location, market, economic climate, and government policy, to name a few.

Public assistance for oral healthcare comes in several forms, and, with ongoing healthcare reform, new modes may be developing that have not existed in the past. Medicare, a federally funded program, provides healthcare coverage for the elderly, and Medicaid provides funding for the indigent. Blocks of federal dollars are usually given to state governments, whose dispersal of these funds must comply with federal guidelines as well as their own additional regulations. Generally, Medicaid and Medicare payments for oral healthcare are minimal and rarely cover preventive treatment. Practice managers need to be familiar with the regulations affecting the specific practice location.

As federal and state funded healthcare programs shrink, increasing numbers of clients do not qualify for government assistance, do not have private insurance, and cannot afford to pay out of pocket for their treatment. These conditions present many challenges in oral healthcare delivery. Someone must provide healthcare for these populations, and every practice is bound to get requests for care from those who are unable to pay. As was the case with public assistance cases, you need to establish policy on how to deal with this, consistent with the practice mission and strategic plan.

Private insurance companies may have a great deal of influence on your fee schedule, especially if your practice is part of a preferred provider organization (PPO), health maintenance organization (HMO), or similar managed care plan. Managed care plans usually control costs by setting strict limits on fees and services. PPOs are administered by establishing a group of preferred providers who agree to provide services to the PPO members at the fee schedule created by the insurance plan. The providers are usually in independent practices and may treat other groups in addition to PPO members. HMOs generally employ their providers and manage their own employees and facilities. There are also combination plans. The PPO or HMO practice generally agrees to treat plan members at discounted fees. In exchange, the practice may receive a flat yearly rate per member covered.

The advantage to the practice of receiving the yearly fee per member is that this cash is received up front, rather than at the time of service. Furthermore, some members may never actually seek treatment in the practice, even though the plan has paid their fee. This may make up for the money lost to the practice through discounting, but it may be impossible to predict what the demand for services will actually be. It is certainly possible for the practice to lose money with such an arrangement. As mentioned previously, this type of managed care, in the absence of quality assurance mechanisms, may lead to an emphasis on quantity rather than quality. The practice cannot realistically agree to provide services at less than cost. Even working with a very narrow profit margin is risky unless you have experience with similar plans and realistic projections of income, expenses, and demand for services for the plan(s) in which the practice participates.

Insurance carriers operating under more traditional plans generally pay some percentage of the fees billed. The percentage varies from carrier to carrier and from procedure to procedure, with some services covered for 100% of the cost, some for as little as 20%, and some not covered at all. The logic of these payment schedules is often obscure. The practice must simply work with them. It is generally possible to submit for preauthorization of costly services, such as crowns. In this case, the dentist submits forms, and usually a radiograph, detailing the treatment plan, and the insurance company then informs its client or the dentist how much of the service it will pay. It is helpful to clients to work with them on preauthorization so that they can better understand the costs of various treatment options. Please note that many professional organizations, including the American Dental Association, have specific policy stating that accepting or tendering rebates or split fees is unethical.

Other groups traditionally receive discounted healthcare: family members, employees, friends, and other health professionals. Practitioners employed in the practice, especially practice owners, will probably expect free oral healthcare for themselves and possibly their families as well. In most practices, all employees receive free treatment and family discounts. Close friends of the practice owners may also expect discounts. Other health professionals usually receive discounted or free treatment. This courtesy may be limited to dentists or physicians, or may be extended to other professionals, such as nurses, hygienists, assistants, and technicians. While this professional courtesy is a common practice, with many marketing advantages, the list of those receiving discounts can be quite long.

The obvious disadvantage to offering free or discounted treatment to family, friends, and colleagues is that the discounts can really affect practice income. The marketing advantage is that these groups are probably an excellent source of referrals, and offering them discounted treatment encourages them to visit and know your practice. If one of your goals is to expand your client base, the referrals can be valuable and may help to offset the loss of income caused by the discounts. Offering free or discounted services to employees and their families has similar marketing benefits. Additionally, this is a benefit that most employees expect. Be sure to promote this as an employment benefit, so that no one takes it for granted. Employees who trust the practice providers enough to seek treatment with them for themselves and their families are also making a personal commitment to the quality of care in the practice.

All fee discounts need to be assessed in terms of their value to the practice. Are the discounts consistent with the mission and plan of the practice? The discount schedule should be prepared in advance, so that no one is caught in an uncomfortable situation when asked about discounts and so that the discounts are applied consistently.

## Incoming Cash Flow

Cash flow can be both positive and negative, income or expense. Good management of incoming cash requires receiving timely payment for services provided and for open invoices.

### THE PAYMENT CYCLE

The payment cycle is the amount of time between billing (invoicing) and receiving payment. Some practices ask for payment at the time of service, either immediately before or after treatment or offer a discount for immediate payment. (There are marketing implications associated with this policy.) In this case, the payment cycle is essentially zero. Fees billed should equal fees collected. Whether or not this is actually the case will depend on how insistent the practice is in enforcing this policy. Collecting for services at the time of treatment is becoming increasingly popular among providers of healthcare because it reduces the payment cycle and reduces billing costs. It may not be as popular with clients, however, and may result in loss of clients.

The payment cycle can be quite long. For a practice that sends bills, it may be a minimum of 45 days. For example, if the practice mails its bills on the first of the month, a client who is seen on the second will not be mailed a bill for another 29 days. Allowing 3–5 additional days for mail processing, 3–5 days for the client to write the check, and another 3–5 days for mail processing, it can easily take 45 days to collect payment, even when the bill has been paid promptly. Some patients may hold the bill for several weeks, or longer, before mailing a payment or may just wait until their next visit to pay. This can have a significant impact on the cash flow of the practice. (See Chapter 3 for further discussion of the time value of money and managing cash flow.) Keeping the payment cycle as short as possible will improve cash flow and this can be critically important.

One way to shorten the payment cycle is to give the client a walk-out statement. Most dental practice computer software can generate walk-out statements. By the time the client is ready to leave the office, the computer can create an up-to-date statement of the client's account. Even if payment is not collected at the time of service, the client as least leaves with a bill (and a detailed treatment record). This shortens the payment cycle by the amount of time it takes to produce and mail the monthly billing, although it does not eliminate the need for monthly billing because not every client pays from the walk-out statement.

## COLLECTION

Some clients don't pay their bills, adding to the difference between the invoices sent and amounts collected. Even if delinquent accounts are eventually collected, costs are associated with the process. If the practice does its own collections, these costs can include phone bills, postage, and legal fees. If the delinquent accounts are turned over to a collection agency, the agency usually takes between 25% and 75% of the amount collected as a fee for its services.

The efficiency of the collection process can make or break a practice. The collection rate should be *at least* 90%. The practice may have to adjust the fees for low-income patients or examine its entire fee schedule if many patients are having difficulty paying. You may also need to modify the billing and/or collection process. These issues will have to be considered during the strategic planning process in accordance with the mission and goals. No matter how high production is, if collections aren't timely, the practice will run into financial problems due to cash flow shortages. Inadequate cash flow can quickly kill a small business.

## INSURANCE PROCESSING

The time required to process insurance claims increases the length of the payment cycle. If the practice waits to receive payment from insurance companies, or clients wait to pay their bills until they receive payment from the insurance company, the accounts can take months to collect. Additionally, if insurance companies don't pay the full amount billed, more time will be spent collecting from the client. Time is also added to the payment cycle if the insurance claims are not processed daily and for mailing in claims and receiving payment. Some computerized practices are using electronic claims processing to reduce mailing time and costs. This procedure usually involves inputting the insurance claims on the practice computer system and then transmitting them to the insurance company's computer by phone. However the claim is filed, the practice has little control over how long the insurance company takes to process the claim, although experience with the carrier is helpful. To reduce errors and speed processing, the person responsible for filing the claims should be familiar with each insurance carrier and its forms and requirements.

### CREDIT CARDS

Credit card fees are charged to businesses by credit card companies. These fees create a difference between the amount billed and the amount collected. Each time a business deposits a credit card payment, the credit card company charges a fee for processing the payment. The charges vary from about 3 to 8%. This means that if a client pays for $78 worth of treatment by credit card, the practice will have to pay a fee between $2.34 and $6.24. What actually happens is that the fees are deducted, by the credit card company, from the amount it pays to the practice account. The fees are a significant source of income for the credit card companies and may cost a practice a significant percentage of its income.

## Quality and Productivity

Quality and productivity are not mutually exclusive. If high quality leads to increased demand for services, and high productivity leads to decreased quality, as is often the case, increasing quality will increase income. It is often difficult for consumers to evaluate the quality of the healthcare they receive. For this reason, the practice must make a continuous effort to inform patients of the quality of services offered and of methods used to monitor and improve quality.

None of the production measures discussed earlier relate specifically to quality. Using a detailed fee schedule will encourage the customization of client services, whereas using cluster fees will tend to emphasize identical service provision for everyone. The latter neglects the important quality aspect of working with each and every client individually. It is probably necessary to have a system of quality assurance in place as well as a system of productivity monitoring. Otherwise, focusing on quantity alone will push the practice toward moving bodies through the doors as fast as possible.

While it is important to monitor productivity, and to strive to maximize it, it is also important not to do so at the expense of quality of care. When quality falls off, productivity will eventually fall off as well, due to loss of market share. Monitoring quality and monitoring productivity must therefore coincide. (See Chapter 5 for a further discussion of quality assurance.)

Consider the example income statement illustrated in Figure 8.1. This DHPC is reasonably profitable and emphasizes high-quality, individualized treatment. In this general practice, most adult patients are given one-hour appointments, many are seen for multiple consecutive periodontal treatment appointments, and plenty of time is allotted for assessment, evaluation, and oral hygiene instructions. While none of these points is a guarantee of quality treatment, there is at least adequate time to provide it.

**Figure 8.1**   *Example income statement*

| | |
|---|---|
| **4th Quarter Income Statement** | |
| **Smallville Dental Group Dental Hygiene Profit Center** | |
| Income from Services | $141,750 |
| Operating Expenses for DHPC | $ 17,010 |
|    Salaries and Benefits | $ 74,098 |
| Operating Expenses due Dental PC | $ 5,016 |
| Operating Earnings | $ 45,627 |
| Depreciation Expense | $ 714 |
| Interest Expense | $ 1,200 |
| Earnings Before Income Tax | $ 41,569 |
| Income Tax Expenses | $ 13,718 |
| Net Income | $ 27,851 |

## Other Sources of Practice Income

A practice may have other sources of income beyond fees for services, including real estate, product sales, and investments. The practice manager may be involved in selecting, recommending, or managing these investments. Sources of real estate income are land or property the practice owns, and may be in addition to the practice site(s) and held only for investment and income value. Income may be generated from rent or may only be equity value in the properties. Not all real estate investments are profitable. A practice with large retained earnings may even consider making real estate investments that deplete cash on hand or offer significant business tax deductions to minimize taxable income and/or retained earnings. A practice may sublease to other businesses some of the space it rents or owns, thereby generating rental income (and expenses).

Some practices may be involved in the sale of goods, usually related to oral healthcare. Some product dealers promote the possibility of generating a significant income for the practice, without using provider time to do so. During the strategic planning process, the practice owners, managers, and employees will have to decide whether product sales are consistent with the practice mission and plan.

Practices may have additional monetary investments that generate income, including pension or retirement plans and such investment vehicles as treasury bills (T bills) or certificates of deposit (CDs) that earn interest. Part of the strategic plan for the practice will involve planning for cash dispersal. A practice that is planning to grow rapidly would be better off investing its cash in expansion (i.e., capital equipment, space, additional personnel) than in T bills or CDs. An older, established practice, in contrast, might have more interest in retirement plans or retained earnings than in spending to promote growth.

## EXPENSES

The type of expenses each practice experiences will depend on its practice setting and mission. The ability of the practice manager to control both production and expenses will also be affected by these variables. While not every practice will be affected by every type of expense discussed in the following sections, many will be similar.

## Payroll, Taxes, and Benefits

As with any service business, salaries and benefits will probably account for most of the operating expenses. Chapters 2 and 7 discussed aspects of human resource management with respect to salaries and benefits. The expenses the practice incurs for salaries and benefits will depend on the numbers and types of employees, as well as the benefits offered. Health insurance and leave benefits alone may amount to as much as 35% of an employee's salary.

In difficult financial times, just making payroll can be quite a challenge. In analyzing the costs of keeping an employee, it is important to look not only at the expenses but at the income as well. What matters to the business will be defined in its mission and goals. If an employee is making a valuable contribution to the practice or profit center, it is probably worth keeping the employee. On the other hand, if the quality of the employee's work is marginal or the costs of employing him exceed the income he generates (directly or indirectly), then the practice needs a more cost-effective employee.

It costs a practice more than just payroll to keep an employee. The employer must make tax contributions equal to a portion of the employee's salary and must also deposit taxes withheld for employees. It is important to note that the Internal Revenue Service (IRS) is very strict about tax payments. Businesses that fall behind in tax payments, especially withholding and payroll taxes, can get into serious trouble quickly. The IRS can freeze, or seize, all the business resources, including bank accounts, property, and capital equipment, to cover back taxes. This can happen quickly and with little regard to due process. For these reasons, managing cash flow is critical for small business survival. Practices that are part of a larger institution with more cash reserves may not have these cash flow worries.

Employee benefits can amount to a significant amount in addition to salary, depending on many factors, including the salary range and benefits received. Private healthcare practices have traditionally been stingy with benefits to reduce these expenses. In a competitive job market, however, it may be necessary to offer a good benefit package in order to attract, and keep, the best employees. An employer located in an area of high unemployment (of healthcare workers) may be able to offer less.

## Debt

Debt may be a significant liability for a dental practice or DHPC because start-up costs are high. This is mostly due to the fact that finished space and equipment are expensive and there are few ways to avoid these expenses. Start-up costs may also include the expense of buying an existing practice, in which case the new owners are also paying for access to the client base. The exact nature of the debt burden will vary according to the situation. Start-up costs are usually financed long term. A practice may also incur new long-term debt when purchasing new capital equipment, such as when setting up a new treatment room or replacing worn-out dental chairs.

Internal profit centers may not be directly responsible for any of the debt expenses but may be assigned a portion of them for space and equipment usage and maintenance. The only way to apportion accurately is to know what the expenses are (including interest) and what portion of the space and equipment is used by the profit center. Do not rely on a guess. These amounts should not be hard to identify.

Until the practice has grown significantly and paid down some of these long-term liabilities, debt payments may amount to as much or more than human resource costs. Realistic initial business planning, sound borrowing, and careful cash flow management are required to handle large debt burdens.

## Rent or Mortgage

Dental hygiene and dental practices may be located in many different types of buildings that the practice owns. These structures vary from converted basements or additions in a residential location, to office parks or office condominium developments, to buildings "built to suit" the practice. Rent or mortgage payments and associated facilities maintenance costs vary considerably from place to place. As the mortgage loan is paid down, the owner's equity in the property increases and the liability decreases. Hopefully, the value of the property and building also increases, though this is not guaranteed. Buildings don't last forever and therefore they do depreciate. The usual schedule for building depreciation is 30 years.

If the practice doesn't own the facility in which it is located, but rents the space, it will have an ongoing liability for rent. Often the terms of commercial leases allow for variable rent amounts. The rent payments may increase (or decrease) each year over the term of the lease. The exact payment schedule will depend on the terms of the lease. A cost that is frequently part of a commercial lease for a practice is the build-out, or finishing, cost. Commercial property often exists as a basic shell and each renter specifies how the rented space is to be finished. Space equipped for special use will generally be more expensive than space in the same facility that is just finished for general office work. For oral healthcare delivery, finishing the space may involve installing electric, plumbing, air, and/or gas lines in the walls, floors, and ceilings. This is costly work. The build-out costs are therefore often spread out over the entire term of the lease to reduce the amount of cash initially invested by the practice owners. One way to reduce the build-out expense is to find a space to lease that has been a dental office in the past and has the plumbing and other necessities already in place.

Mortgage or rent costs won't apply if the practice is located in a building that it owns outright (all loans paid). In some public health settings, such as schools, there may not be a rent or mortgage charge. Even in the cases where there is no direct expense for rent or mortgage, the practice will incur facilities usage and maintenance costs.

## Usage and Maintenance

The costs for usage and maintenance depend on the type of facility in which the practice is located. Commercial properties are often categorized by the amount of finish and service associated with the property. The most common categories are warehouse, office, research and development (R&D), and full service. Warehouse spaces are large, open buildings, more than one story high in the interior, and completely unfinished. These spaces are generally suitable only for storage or industrial purposes. Office space is generally located in one-story buildings. The business leasing office or warehouse space is generally responsible for all facility maintenance, including utilities, insurance, and the heating, ventilation, and air conditioning system (HVAC). All the business gets from the landlord is the shell, finished to comply with the terms of the lease agreement. R&D space is a combination of office and warehouse space, usually with finished offices in front and open bay (or warehouse space) with loading docks in the rear. Maintenance terms for R&D space are usually the same as those for warehouse or office space.

Full-service buildings are fully finished office buildings, usually multistory. The cost of leasing space in full-service buildings usually includes utilities, janitorial services for the common areas (lobby, halls, etc.), building security (if it exists), and often janitorial service for the office space as well. In multistory buildings, the hours of building access are often limited. A full-service building is typically open for use only during regular business hours, but a smaller number may be open evenings and Saturdays. During the off hours, there may not be HVAC service. These terms and conditions will be delineated in the lease. Usage and maintenance expenses can be significant, especially if you have old equipment or are located in an older facility.

Utilities, including phone, power (electric, gas, or both), and water are part of usage costs. Expert advice is often available through the utility companies on ways to manage costs. You may have a number of options available for long-distance phone service. Adjust the expenses as best you can, without investing too much management time. In the case of a financial crisis, you can often make special payment arrangements with the utility companies if you contact them as soon as you realize you may have a problem.

## Insurance

Insurance costs also vary considerably from one location to another and from one practice setting to another. Insurance costs incurred by a dental practice or DHPC will be for property coverage (fire, flood, etc.), general liability (if someone slips and falls, for example), and professional liability (malpractice). The insurance rates for property and general liability are affected by the location and the nature of the business and its claims record.

Professional liability insurance may be associated with an entire practice or with individual practitioners or both. Large institutions, especially, may have group liability coverage. Malpractice insurance for dental hygienists is relatively inexpensive, especially compared to the cost of similar coverage for dentists or physicians. There is little variation in the cost of professional liability coverage for dental hygienists. Rates are similar regardless of supervision requirements, scope of practice, or practice setting, and are currently under $250 per year. The cost of liability coverage for dentists may be 10 to 100 times greater and will depend on the type of practice and the dentist's claims record.

## Supplies and Inventory

Controlling supply costs is frequently a concern. Supplies used in the DHPC may include all types of disposables (masks, gloves, prophy angles, plastic covers, gauze, autoclave bags, etc.), x-ray film, polishing paste, various types of fluoride treatments, home care supplies, and so on. In addition to these, supplies used in dental profit centers may include more costly items such as impression and restorative materials and surgical supplies. There are also pieces of equipment, mostly hand instruments such as mirrors, curettes, and carvers, which have short life spans (less than three years) and are considered supplies for accounting purposes. Many practices will have expenses for educational materials (handouts, brochures, slides, posters, tapes, etc.).

Supplies cost money. You don't want the practice to have an excessive amount of cash tied up in supply inventories that are just sitting around not being used. Additionally, many of the supplies used in oral healthcare, such as drugs and fluorides, have limited life spans. If you overstock, you may have to throw away ("waste") expired products. You want to have the necessary supplies on hand when you need them, but not too long before that. The best method for controlling supply inventories is to keep records of receipt of shipments and rate of usage of supplies. You will then have the data you need to predict your supply needs accurately. If you don't keep detailed records in an easy-to-use format, you will be left guessing at purchasing decisions. The worst case would be to get caught short of critical supplies and cause a decrease in quality or production.

Managing suppliers is an art form. Purchasing management is a specialized field and large businesses and institutions may have professional purchasing managers. Small businesses will not have these resources. This may be an advantage, in that purchasing and inventory systems can be smaller, simpler, and more responsive, a position that even the largest manufacturers are trying to emulate. The ideal is to work with a limited number of suppliers (about five or six) who are totally responsive to your needs. Choosing the best suppliers involves more than just getting the best price. You also need a cost-effective system where you receive competitive pricing (not always the lowest, not the highest), good customer service, order, delivery, and billing schedules that fit your requirements. It will take time and adjustments to streamline the purchasing system, and it will also require attention and adjustment from time to time. The person managing purchasing doesn't have to be the practice or profit center manager. In a small practice, this may be the only option, but in a large practice there may be other personnel with an interest or expertise in purchasing.

Purchasing hand instruments can be managed through your regular purchasing system, with attention given to the requirements of individual practitioners. Giving employees control over their own instrument selection can be an effective motivator. As discussed in previous chapters, people are motivated by being empowered to make their own choices about how to do their jobs. Instrument selection seems like a minor issue, but it can be very important to individuals. Give each practitioner a quarterly or yearly instrument budget. Just be sure that the practitioners understand the budget within which they have to work.

Managers are always concerned about controlling costs. The short-term solution may appear to be to purchase the cheapest goods available, but there are costs associated with supply and instrument failures. For example, using low-cost, low-quality restorative materials may lead to complaints, loss of clients, and decreased provider productivity. Similarly, some DHPCs use retipped scalers and curettes to save money. Unfortunately, retipped instruments are much more likely to break and are frequently too bulky to be used effectively subgingivally. Saving a few hundred dollars on instruments over the years will not make up for the costs of just one malpractice suit brought by a client who suffers an injury from a broken curette. Decreasing the efficiency of dental hygienists' work by forcing them to use retipped instruments affects the productivity of the DHPC. When making purchasing decisions, consider the total impact of product quality on other areas of your business.

## Temporary Help

Occasions will arise when practitioners are unavailable at the last minute. Your alternatives will be to cancel clients, hire temporary help (temps), or (in the case of a missing assistant) run behind schedule. The costs associated with canceling clients or running late include not just the loss of income for one day, but also the loss of client goodwill. Furthermore, clients will not appreciate your being late or canceling appointments at the last minute. If this is a frequent annoyance, they may choose another practice. If you can be late or cancel at the last minute, clients may feel that they can also.

Costs associated with using temporary practitioners (usually hygienists) include more than agency fees. Loss of client goodwill may occur. Patients may not be satisfied with seeing a practitioner they do not know and have not selected. Most will be happy to be treated by a temp if given a choice (as far in advance as possible). The temp must also be able to meet the quality assurance standards of the practice. If the practitioner you replace with a temp is on salary or has applicable leave benefits, you will have to pay the regular employee as well as the temp. Because the need for temporary help usually arises unexpectedly, the practice manager should do research and cost effectiveness analysis in advance to determine the best methods to use. In some cases it may be more cost effective to cancel a day's clients and in other cases it may be better to use temporary help.

## Marketing

All practices incur some direct costs for marketing. Managing marketing and advertising is discussed in detail in Chapter 10. If a practice chooses to advertise, there will be specific costs for this. The DHPC, or other profit centers, may be assigned a portion of the advertising costs for the practice setting. Decreasing marketing costs may be an effective means of decreasing short-term expenses, but keep in mind that marketing is keeping the practice going by keeping clients coming through the door. Eliminating all marketing will be a failure in the long run.

## Outgoing Cash Flow

Cash flows out of a practice when expenses are paid. Careful management of outgoing cash flow involves making timely payment with available resources. While a practice needs to meet its financial obligations on time to maintain good relations with employees and creditors, this does not mean that every invoice should be paid the day it is received. The practice must always meet payroll and tax payments on time, but creditors should be managed by priority.

Cash flow projections are used for this planning. Cash flow projections predict the income and expenses expected in the future (usually the next 30–90 days). There are various ways to prepare cash flow statements. The easiest is to use a computer that contains the practice's financial records. Many standard software packages include cash flow reporting. If these resources are not available, cash flow projections can be prepared manually. Income projections are based on current accounts receivable (all open accounts), sorted by due date (and may need to be adjusted by data on when the account is expected to be paid). There is also some guesswork involved, especially long term, as it is not always possible to predict exactly what the practice income will be in the future. Historical data may help— for example, some months may be notoriously slow. Expense projections are based on current accounts payable, plus an estimate of usual expenses or planned additional expenses. As with income projections, guesswork is involved.

Many businesses, especially small businesses, run into situations where, although there is adequate income invoiced, or controlled expenses, there is not enough cash in the bank to meet all outstanding financial obligations at once. Cash flow projections are used to predict these situations and avoid or control them. If you project a cash shortage, you must also plan to manage it without losing clients or alienating suppliers. On the expense side, this means planning expenses and payments carefully so that adequate cash is on hand when payments are due. Some businesses cope with cash flow problems by establishing with a bank a line of credit, or a preapproved amount that can be drawn on at any time. It is short-term financing, with a short payback period, whose terms are set when the line is established. One example of using a line of credit in private practice might be when large insurance payments are slow and there is insufficient cash to meet payroll. You can draw on the line of credit to meet payroll and repay the loan when your payment for services is received.

## UNDERSTANDING PROFITABILITY

The preceding discussion has outlined some sources of income and possible expenses for dental and dental hygiene practice. Profit is income minus expenses. In not-for-profit practice settings, such as public health facilities and some hospitals, profitability is not an issue, although managers are responsible for working within the established budget. In for-profit settings, of course, profitability is important.

As an example, consider the profitability of a DHPC. Chapter 6 discussed the reasons for treating the provision of dental hygiene services as a separate profit center. This can be handled solely as a financial matter, without affecting actual clinical services, and involves keeping separate financial records for the DHPC. The DHPC can use any convenient accounting method. Using the same methods as the practice setting will be most efficient. In the long run, the most cost-effective tool for maintaining financial records is almost always a computer. The financial statements generated by the DHPC will be similar to those discussed in Chapter 3. Figure 8.1 is an example income statement for the DHPC in the Smallville Dental Group.

For this example, the DHPC is defined as follows. The Smallville Group is located in a state with indirect supervision requirements. A dentist must be present at all times when dental hygiene patients are being treated. After examining the year-end financial statements (presented in Chapter 3) and reviewing the strategic plan, the owner of the Smallville Group realized that the dental hygiene portion of her practice needed to be modified.

During the strategic planning process, the decision was made to create a dental hygiene profit center and to change to an accelerated dental hygiene practice. The current dental hygienist was qualified to manage the newly created DHPC. A second dental hygiene treatment room was set up and a dental hygiene assistant was hired and trained. The hygienist and assistant worked out of two treatment rooms. Most adult patients were scheduled for one-hour appointments, as they had been in the past. The hygienist and assistant saw patients 35 hours per week and spent five hours per week on management and administrative duties and staff meetings.

Figure 8.1 is the year-end income statement for the DHPC. It reflects the operations of the DHPC after one full year of accelerated dental hygiene practice. This income statement is for the DHPC only. In the Smallville Group, the DHPC is an integral part of the dental practice, so the year-end financial reports for the practice would include the amounts from the DHPC. The report presented in Figure 8.1 would be for internal use only.

The gross income from services for the DHPC for the year ($141,750) was generated by treating an average of nine patients per day, at an average fee of $70 per client, assuming the DHPC operated 50 weeks per year. The accelerated practice was able to accommodate all of the new patients who entered the practice that year, many of whom needed initial periodontal therapy in the DHPC. The average fee per client may decrease as a larger percentage of patients move into the maintenance phase of their treatment. Fees for the dentist's examinations were credited directly to the dental profit center. Patients who were seen briefly by the dentist during the dental hygiene appointment were not charged and the DHPC was not charged for the dentist's time for these cases.

The operating expenses have been divided into two categories: the DHPC and the dental profit center. The expenses of the DHPC are 12% of the gross, mostly for supplies and instruments, but also including insurance. The operating expenses due the dental profit center include rent ($15 per square foot for 200 feet for both hygiene treatment rooms), 15% of the receptionist's time, and 20% of the utility and maintenance charges.

The salaries and benefits for the DHPC (the assistant and hygienist) are listed separately to simplify analyzing these costs during the first year of accelerated practice. The hygienist's salary is $38,000 and the assistant's salary is $18,000 per year. Other benefits, including health insurance, leave, and professional development fees (for dues, CE, etc.), are 20% of salary. This figure may be low, but the employees are highly motivated by the amount of responsibility and autonomy they have and the recognition they receive. They also receive a 5% year-end bonus on gross income above the target level of $110,000. The DHPC pays just under 11% in payroll taxes, unemployment taxes, and workman's compensation. The total of salaries and benefits amounts to about 52% of gross income. This amount is higher than some practice management firms suggest, but, as you will see, the overall profitability of the DHPC is excellent, so this formula is working well for this practice. The total year-end operating earnings are $45,627.

The DHPC has been assigned the total cost of $20,000 for equipping the second dental hygiene treatment room, even though the actual liability was incurred by the practice. The depreciation and interest charges for this debt are charged to the DHPC, making its before tax income $41,569. The income tax expense on this amount is also charged to the DHPC.

The net income (bottom line) for the DHPC for the year is $27,851. If the change in the DHPC led to a 20% increase in income for the Smallville Group (as compared to the amounts in Figure 3.3), the gross income from services for the entire practice would increase to $795,600 and net income would increase to approximately $55,650. The DHPC would therefore account for 18% of the gross, and 50% of the net, income.

The Smallville Group has a profitable DHPC. The net income is about 20% of the gross income. Also, the Smallville DHPC is earning a higher than average percentage of the total practice net income, due in part to the fact that the dentist-owner's salary and benefits, which she keeps relatively high, are charged to the expenses of the dental profit center. This makes it appear to be less profitable than the DHPC, where salaries are lower.

The profit generated by the DHPC may be retained by the practice or may be reinvested in the DHPC. The DHPC might use its retained earnings for capital equipment purchases, for marketing, or for whatever purposes are indicated by the strategic plan.

## *Summary*

Good financial management is important for survival. Even not-for-profit practices must operate within budget. In oral healthcare delivery, income is generated mostly from providing services and many methods are available for tracking that production. The method of choice will depend on the mission of the practice. There are many ways to structure a fee schedule, mostly applicable to for-profit practices. A key to financial survival in for-profit settings is managing cash flow. While cash flow involves both income and expenses, management is usually easier when cash income is abundant.

The connections between quality and productivity cannot be overlooked. These two concepts are closely related in oral healthcare, to the point that one may not exist for long without the other.

There are also an unlimited number of possible expenses for any oral health-care practice. The practice's profit orientation, mission, and market will influence which expenses apply. Regardless of all these factors, every manager will be concerned with controlling expenses.

Profit is income minus expenses. In not-for-profit settings, zero profit may be acceptable, but continued negative profit (operating loss) may lead to loss of funding. Managers of for-profit practices will be concerned with maintaining a positive bottom line, consistent with the practice's mission.

## Review Questions

1. Describe two methods of tracking productivity in the DHPC.
2. Describe two methods of tracking productivity in a DPC.
3. Discuss the advantages and disadvantages of using detailed fee schedules.
4. Define the payment cycle.
5. Discuss three factors that influence the length of the payment cycle.
6. Discuss three ways to reduce the length of the payment cycle.
7. State one reason for achieving timely fee collections.
8. Describe six possible expenses for dental hygiene or dental practice.
9. Define profit.
10. Refer to the financial statements presented in Chapter 3. Is the Smallville Dental Group profitable?
11. Define a hypothetical profit center and create an income statement for it.
12. Analyze an existing practice and describe ways in which it would be useful for the practice to separate its profit centers.

## SUGGESTED READING

Gumpert, D. E. (1990). *How to really create a successful business plan.* Boston: Inc. Publishing.

Kroll, L. (1980). *A room with no window.* Torrance: Author.

Livingstone, J. L. (1992). *The portable MBA in finance and accounting.* New York: John Wiley & Sons.

Simini, J. P. (1990). *Balance sheet basics for non-financial managers.* New York: John Wiley & Sons.

Thomas, R. D. (1987). *Career directions for dental hygienists.* New Jersey: Career Directions Press.

Tracy, J. A. (1989). *How to read a financial report.* New York: John Wiley & Sons.

Woodall, I., & Bentley, J. M. (1983). *Legal, ethical and management aspects of the dental care system* (2nd ed.). St. Louis: C.V. Mosby.

Wright, R. O. (1990). *A little bit at a time: Secrets of productive quality.* Berkeley: Ten Speed Press.

# CHAPTER 9

# Marketing Oral Healthcare Services

## Objectives

After reading this chapter and completing the review questions, the reader should be able to:

- State the importance of market research.
- Describe a client database.
- Describe marketing price, position, and promotion.
- Describe the role of public relations in marketing oral healthcare delivery.
- Describe some of the ethical considerations involved in "selling" healthcare.
- Describe the role of advertising in marketing oral healthcare delivery.
- Describe the process of marketing oral healthcare delivery.

Marketing can take place in any practice setting, although it is most closely associated with for-profit, private practices. Marketing oral healthcare services can improve more than profit. Marketing can increase access to and utilization of healthcare services, can promote preventive health behaviors, and ultimately can improve health.

## MARKET RESEARCH

All marketing should begin with research. Market research examines the demographics, interests, and marketing variables of the potential client pool. Information gathered from market research can be used to develop new products or services, to modify existing products or services, or to identify new market segments. Market research need not be expensive, esoteric, or professional. You may well have the information and ability within your practice to perform and update your market research on a regular basis. Use the information gathered through market research to develop your marketing plan and define the price, position, and promotion for your various services.

## Client Database

Client records are the best source of marketing information. Clinicians and business personnel regularly collect and update client information, either during regular visits or through mailings. If your practice uses a computer for billing and record keeping, you can customize your client database to provide the information required for your market research. Computerized information is easier to sort than paper files, but a computer is not magic. A well-organized manual record-keeping system can function just as well as a computerized one, especially in a small practice. The key to success, to timely information, is to continually gather and update relevant information.

Gather as much information in your client database as possible. You will be limited by storage space (either office space or space on your computer's hard disk), personnel time, and the patience of your clients to answer questions. For each client, as a minimum, you should have basic demographic data, such as name, address (with zip code), phone number(s), and birth date. Other items for adults may include business address, occupation, highest level of education, sports, hobbies, community activities, names of spouse or significant other, children and other dependents, and individual characteristics, such as disabilities or special achievements. Other items for children may include school, grade level, names of parents or guardians, siblings, sports or academic interests, hobbies, and individual characteristics.

## Other Sources of Marketing Information

There are additional sources of marketing information, beginning with the public library. A reference librarian can provide a world of information on sources of local facts, not just about population demographics, but about other areas of special interest as well.

The importance of research in marketing planning cannot be overemphasized. Guesswork will not produce accurate predictions of market niches, client interests and potential markets. You must conduct research to gather facts, a task that may be as simple as sorting your existing client database by age or asking your local librarian to provide a list of area elementary schools and numbers of students enrolled. Remember that your market research is for internal use and does not have to meet the rigorous research standards used for publication.

Marketing planning can be a part of your overall strategic planning. During regular planning sessions, identify the information you'll need for marketing planning and incorporate the necessary data collection procedures into normal operations. Feed back market research data into the planning process so that your plan is responsive to the environment, clients, and potential clients. The price, position, and promotional strategies you develop for marketing should be integral to the achievement of the overall plan.

## PRICE, POSITION, PROMOTION

The market *position* of services is often defined by the *price*. For example, if your for-profit practice offers very low or discount fees, you'll attract a different type of client than will a practice that charges premium fees. Clients most interested in low fees might be low-income groups who would accept some compromises in comfort or elegance to save money. A nonprofit practice, such as a public health clinic, is defined by being free or low cost. Marketing efforts in a public health practice might be geared toward attracting clients by informing the public of the availability of services or by *promoting* positive health behaviors. The market positions of a discount for-profit private practice and a public health clinic would differ. The discount practice might position itself as a low-cost alternative for many groups, even those with the funds or insurance to cover more expensive treatment. The public health clinic might have a more limited market, as defined by its mission or sponsoring agency. A public health practice might even be restricted to treating only those clients meeting the guidelines of the sponsoring agency, such as financial need. Other examples of market position for dental or dental hygiene practice might include marketing services for families, the elderly, federal employees (or employees of a particular industry or business), or groups with special needs, such as the physically handicapped or medically compromised.

Successful marketing depends on carefully defining a particular market segment or niche, customizing your services to suit the needs of that group, and *promoting* the specificity of your market position. For example, rather than *promote* your practice to children, you would probably be more successful if you segmented your marketing efforts to appeal to specific groups, such as families of preschoolers, high school students, and little league players.

Market share is a term used frequently in marketing. It describes the percentage of a particular market niche served by your practice. For example, if you position your practice as one that serves retired persons, you would determine the total population of retirees (data from the census, at your local library) in your geographic area (probably by ZIP code). The number of retirees who are your clients (data from your client database) divided by the total population of retirees is the percentage of the retiree market your practice serves—your market share. Use the specific market share information to set objectives and to evaluate the success of your marketing programs.

## PUBLIC RELATIONS

Marketing functions have previously been discussed as public relations, sales, and advertising. We will now consider each of these functions as they relate to oral healthcare delivery.

Any given practice may pursue a variety of public relations activities, depending on its mission, plans, and environment. It is important to keep in mind that public relations activities are frequently long range and that their efficacy is often difficult to evaluate. For these and other reasons, it is often helpful to pursue a number of activities simultaneously. Public relations activities may be directed to the community, to professional groups, or internally, to staff members.

## The Community

The public at large generally expects healthcare providers and practices to provide public service, and professionals have an obligation to share their expertise with their communities. Community service projects can take almost any form, not just related to oral healthcare, but to healthcare in general, and to other community needs as well.

The purpose of community service is not to promote your practice, but to serve your community. The benefits may not be direct or immediate, but the work you, and other staff members, do in the community will be rewarded in many, often unexpected ways. The short-term and most immediate benefit to the practice is that all of the employees involved in community service projects will be recognized by other service-minded individuals and consumers. This will also help to establish your practice position in community leadership, and possibly also in business leadership. Clients looking for healthcare providers might have more confidence in someone they know is volunteering to help others.

Beyond the immediate results of recognition and leadership, community service involvement can provide many valuable business, personal, and professional contacts. Community service is a way of networking with others, outside your own field. Creating a public image as a group of concerned, involved individuals may also help to prevent public relations disasters in time of trouble. This is not an endorsement of influence pedaling, corruption, or favor swapping, but eventually the good you do is recognized, often in unexpected ways. For example, services that you provide through the local hospice or homeless shelter will probably not directly bring new patients into your private practice. However, through such work you may meet or be of service to someone who is eventually able to be of help to you or your practice when you really need it. Also, most of those in healthcare have gotten involved in their field to be able to make a real contribution to the betterment of people's lives and health, and community service frequently provides the most personally satisfying experiences you will have in your entire career.

Beyond public service, additional public relations vehicles are available to you to communicate with the community(ies) you serve. You might consider producing a newsletter, either in-house, if you have the staff expertise and computer equipment available, or by subcontracting to a local business. Most print shops can give advice on newsletter production. In larger communities there are often small businesses that offer desktop publishing and newsletter production as one of their services. If none exist in your area, you might consider encouraging a staff member or client to start a small business of this type. There are also businesses that specialize in producing newsletters or copy (articles) for dental practices. These services usually offer their clients template newsletters on a regular basis. They supply the copy, art, and sometimes the layout, and you add a few names, pictures, and the like specific to your practice, and have your local printer prepare your copies. Some of these newsletter services will produce and mail your entire newsletter for you.

The newsletter need not be produced on a regular basis. It could be quarterly or yearly, as fits the marketing plan. If you have specific market niche information about your clients, you might want to tailor issues to certain markets, such as teens or parents, and just mail a newsletter to those individuals. Your newsletters may go to existing clients or to potential clients, but remember to customize the message for the target audience. What you have to offer existing clients may not be of particular interest to potential clients, who need information on selecting a practitioner and on what services you offer that meet their needs.

As with other forms of communication, be sure that your newsletter conveys the image you want. For example, if you are a very casual, easy-going practice, and you know that this is what your target market is looking for, your newsletter should reflect this. It should be informal, use simple typefaces, include pictures and illustrations, be printed on colored paper, and use casual language. On the other hand, if your practice caters to a more formal, intellectual crowd, your newsletters to them should be more formal, use black type on white paper, use more advanced vocabulary, perhaps include charts or graphs, and cover topics of interest to that group. If your practice serves both groups, you should probably produce more than one newsletter, though perhaps not for every issue. You may only have the resources to touch each group once a year, but the more you reach out to your clients, the more they will respond to you. Additionally, solicit feedback from your existing clients on the newsletters they receive and ask new clients to comment if they mention receiving one of your newsletters. In this way, you can continually improve the newsletters. Newsletters can be an efficient, cost-effective method of reaching specific target groups with specific messages.

Another method of reaching your community members is to offer open houses and tours. For an open house, open your facility for informal visits or a party, when no clients are scheduled. You might want to tie in your open house with a holiday, for example, a sugar-free costume party at Halloween or in the spring for clients or neighbors in your office building, or a tobacco-free theme for the opening of baseball season. December is always a good month for an open house, perhaps in conjunction with the office party. Doing *all* of these could get expensive and use up a significant amount of production time, but an open house offers a valuable opportunity to invite new and existing clients to visit your facility and get to know the staff in a casual setting.

What children often fear most about visits to healthcare providers is the unknown. They will be much more relaxed for treatment appointments if they have had an initial visit to your office when no treatment was performed. You can, of course, do this on an individual basis, and for phobic adults, this may be the best approach. It is often possible, however, to arrange for groups of children, from local schools or preschools, to visit for an organized tour. Tours may also be arranged as part of your other community service projects. While it is good for visitors to get a feel for regular office activities, you must be sensitive to the confidentiality of your clients' records and treatment. It is probably best not to schedule tours during treatment times and certainly not to bring tour groups into a treatment room where a client is being seen without the client's permission. Client and staff records should not be accessible to visitors at any time.

## Your Clients

Your clients are members of the community at large, and you might also consider them a special community themselves. Every client who visits your practice has invested time and expense to be there. If you want them to remain loyal, it is probably not enough to just provide them with high-quality oral health services. You need to take every opportunity to acknowledge that you appreciate that they have chosen your practice, using methods that will vary according to the nature of your practice and interests of your clients. The following discussion covers a number of methods that have generally proven successful for a variety of dental and dental hygiene practices. All or none of these may be applicable to your practice. Choose your activities based on your clients and your resources.

New clients should be welcomed to your practice. You may do this by putting a "welcome to our practice" sign on the wall or client bulletin board in the reception area, listing the names of all the new clients you are expecting that day. Another successful welcome method is to send each new client a "thank you for visiting us" note after their first visit.

It is unfortunate, but true, that clients often experience pain associated with their visits to you (before, during, or after). It is important to help clients deal with pain as much as possible (beyond providing adequate pain control measures). One approach is to call clients who came in pain, had pain during the visit, or may have pain later. The person who treated them (dentist or hygienist) should give them a call after the close of business or the next day to inquire how they are doing. This may also apply to clients who had very long appointments, or were given new appliances, crowns, or bridges. Phone follow-up within 24 hours with surgery patients is especially important.

If your practice is charging premium fees, clients expect premium service. You may choose to have small gifts on hand to reward clients who have had long or difficult procedures. It has become standard to offer small toys or stickers for children. Other items (for adults or children) might include flowers or balloons, imprinted giveaways such as pens, magnets, mugs, or key chains. Recipes and other informational pieces are sometimes popular. Choose items that are consistent with the practice image and appeal to *clients*, not the staff person placing the order. Whenever possible, include your practice logo and name on the giveaway items so that each item becomes a marketing piece, as well as a reward.

Photographs are well received. You may photograph your clients at regular maintenance visits and display the pictures in an album or on a bulletin board. Children respond especially well to photos. Old photos can be placed in the client records. It is nice to see an 18-year-old who has been a client since he was 2, but producing a photo of his first visit is really special. Photographs can be equally important for adults, many of whom do not appreciate the impact of their treatment until they see before and after pictures. With client permission, the before and after shots can be used as important marketing tools for explaining treatment options and effects to other clients. Photos can be used to document cases for publication or discussion with colleagues, or may be sent with referral, thank-you letters, or treatment summaries. Your before and/or after pictures can tell a colleague volumes about a case you are referring or have treated. The investment in photographic equipment and training will more than pay for itself over time. Additionally, this is an activity in which assistants, hygienists, and dentists can become involved, and may provide rewarding opportunities for staff development.

Your reception area will be the first part of the practice that clients encounter. (Notice that the current terminology is *reception area*, not waiting room.) Different groups have varying time sense—an unacceptably long wait for a member of one group may be perfectly acceptable to a member of another. Adjust your scheduling to suit the majority of your clients. If, for example, you see many emergencies, or you can anticipate that your clients may have long waits, they may appreciate a television in the reception area.

It has long been the trend in office design to put the receptionist behind a wall or high counter, sometimes with only a small window for communication with clients. Consider the message this arrangement sends clients. It does not convey an open, caring, welcoming attitude. The receptionist should not be walled off from the clients. Instead, use a small, nearby business office not open directly into the reception area or a private business office(s) for sensitive or confidential work.

The reception area is an excellent place to present your clients with pertinent information. Use it accordingly. What you choose to display and have available will depend on the interests of your clients and your marketing plan. Clients are focused on oral health when they visit, so the reception area is an excellent place to position health messages, for example, about smoking cessation, benefits of fluorides and sealants, and the need for blood pressure and cholesterol screening. Don't display everything at once or have too many messages. Reading materials and displays can be simple and direct; clients who want more information should be encouraged to ask questions. Change the displays regularly to cut down on clutter and keep the information new. The reception area can also be used to display your marketing pieces, such as before and after photos of your cases, awards, or distinctions earned by the staff. Again, keep the message simple and the room uncluttered.

The reception area should, as a minimum, contain up-to-date reading material of interest to your clients. Magazines are usually most convenient. Keep the issues current and choose magazines that will be of interest to the various groups you serve (including children, if applicable). You may also use books or posters or have videotape programs available.

You can choose from a variety of marketing activities to acknowledge or reward patients. Choose activities that appeal to your clients, for example, toys or video games in the reception area of pediatric or family practices. Some practices offer complementary (sugar-free) beverages. If you cater to businesspeople during working hours, they will appreciate brief waits, a quiet reception area with room to work, outlets for their laptop computers, and occasional access to your office copier.

Dental hygienists can be very effective in marketing dental services. They generally spend more time talking with clients than any other employee and can use this time to discuss clients' health and oral health needs. Dental hygienists often do a great deal of data collection and assessment. Identifying problem areas to clients during data collection provides opportunities for dialog regarding client needs such as further treatment and referral to other practitioners.

The marketing possibilities for targeting your clients are unlimited. Base your choices on client input, limited tests, and past success. Keep testing new ideas. Even activities that were initially successful may lose their effectiveness over time.

## Other Professionals

The opportunities to interact with other healthcare professionals are numerous, and each should be viewed, at least partially, as public relations activities. Professional interaction should not be limited to practice owners only, but should include all staff members whenever possible. For example, referrals to a dental practice often come from contacts dental hygienists make through the dental hygiene association.

Healthcare professionals can be one of your best sources of new clients and will be your primary source if you are in a specialty practice. You need specific marketing, not just public relations, strategies to reach this group, and the possibilities are endless. You may get new ideas from colleagues, staff, the media, or clients. Traditional PR activities include thank-you letters to those professionals, friends, and clients for referrals, as well as gifts and other acknowledgments to those who refer to you frequently. Additionally, any healthcare professional who refers a client to your practice should receive a timely follow-up letter from you outlining your treatment (planned and/or completed). The client should also be returned to the referring professional to continue treatment there as needed, unless ethical considerations prevent this. The quickest way to lose your referral base is to "steal" clients by not returning them to the referral. The importance of these thank-you letters and treatment summaries cannot be overlooked. Such communications have become an industrywide standard, and no professional practice should ignore these simple courtesies.

In the course of your community service activities, you will probably have ample opportunities to interact with other healthcare professionals. If you do not encounter them, your community may be suffering from a lack of involvement of healthcare professionals. Seek them out and encourage them to join your community service activities.

There may be services you can provide, free of charge, for other practices, as part of your PR activities. For example, if you or another staff member is or becomes a certified cardiopulmonary resuscitation (CPR) instructor, you can offer CPR certification programs for the practices that refer to you most often. This may also be a good method of initial contact with other community groups, such as day-care centers or long-term care facilities. Additionally, if you have specialized equipment, such as a phase contrast microscope or panoral machine, you may want to accept referrals for these services only, at a minimum cost, as a service to your referring practices. Finally, the healthcare practitioners you refer to should refer to you.

If they are not, find out why. There may be some problem with your practice that you are unaware of that no one will mention unless you push them to explain.

Practitioners who refer to your practice will likewise expect you to refer to them. You do have an ethical obligation to refer your clients to competent practitioners, and your recommendations will reflect on your practice. Apply any available quality assurance measures to the practices to which you refer clients, and try, diplomatically, to help the other practice improve if you discover a problem. If this is not possible, stop referring your clients to them. If you are openly critical of other providers' services when speaking to clients or others, you may risk legal action. Choose your words carefully (this applies to all staff members). Be sure you have facts to prove your claims of poor quality or incompetence. It may be simpler to just omit names from your referral list rather than offer details. In most cases, it is probably illegal to systematically exclude certain practices from referrals (based on race, gender, age, religious preferences, etc.), either in your practice only, or in conjunction with others.

Every staff member should be an active member of some professional group. Association involvement should not be overlooked. Not only will you and the rest of the staff make some of your most valuable professional contacts through participating in your professional association, you may make some of your best friends that way. Additionally, it is the obligation of every professional to exchange ideas and information with colleagues. Association membership is not only important for public relations, it is a key element of staff development and service activities.

## Your Staff

Public relations activities are most often thought of as directed from the practice outward, but internal public relations is just as important to the practice's long-term viability. If the practice is to reach its potential, you will need a motivated, involved staff. Think of staff development activities in terms of being an internal public relations campaign.

There are many ways to approach internal PR, and the best methods will vary depending on the type of practice and its mission. For example, in a practice with a large staff of ten or more, a staff newsletter can be an effective communication vehicle. The newsletter can be the responsibility of one person with an interest in desktop publishing, or the responsibility may rotate among all the staff or departments. If you implement a staff newsletter, solicit feedback. If the general consensus is that the newsletter is "stupid" or "a waste of time" or "too much work," change your strategies.

An alternative or adjunct to the newsletter is the staff bulletin board. For a small staff, the bulletin board is more practical than a newsletter. It should be in the staff break area, not in client areas, although there may be a client bulletin board as well. The staff bulletin board (or newsletter) should contain information about staff development activities, such as who attended which continuing education courses, as well the attendee's report of what was learned. Additional items might include personal announcements (weddings, births, etc.) or photos. What is included depends on the staff, but it is best to keep the contents positive. Negative comments should not be suppressed, but a staff newsletter or bulletin is not the best vehicle for addressing problems. They should be handled at staff, individual, or informal meetings.

Recognition of accomplishments, no matter how minor, should be included in the internal PR program. Include professional and, if appropriate, personal items. For example, post certificates of appreciation received by staff members for participation in community or professional groups. Most groups recognize birthdays, with a lunch or cake. Group achievements, such as the completion of a major project or reaching an objective, should be recognized with awards and appropriate celebration. The possibilities are unlimited. Just be sure that all positive accomplishments are publicly recognized.

## SALES

Providing healthcare services is not like selling cars, but the marketing activities of a healthcare practice are analogous to selling a product. The client is the customer and what you are selling is services. If no one is buying, you are out of business, no matter how high the quality of your services. Each time a client visits your practice for treatment, you are making a sale. McDonald's fast-food restaurants place signs on their exit doors that say, "We know you had a choice and we're glad you chose McDonald's." Similarly, for every visit to your practice, a client has made a choice to come to you. Clients might have chosen to go elsewhere or not have treatment. Appreciate and acknowledge your clients' choice to seek treatment with your practice. Your staff is not doing them a favor in treating them; don't make them feel that you are.

Ethical considerations are involved in "selling" healthcare services. While every effort should be made to explain all possible treatment options to a client, including the dentist's or hygienist's professional opinion of which treatment option is most viable, it is highly unethical to promote unnecessary treatment. Unfortunately, the line between necessary and unnecessary is often unclear. If too much emphasis is placed on "selling" in a healthcare practice, the likelihood increases that unnecessary services will be performed or that clients will be encouraged to choose treatment options beyond their budgets. Balance the need to market your services with ethical considerations, and be consistent with the practice's philosophy and mission.

A classic method of increasing sales volume is to increase the average transaction price. To return to a fast-food example, if each client who visits your restaurant to buy a $1 hamburger is also sold a $1 bag of french fries, your sales revenue will double without requiring any investment in new equipment or personnel (assuming french fries were already on the menu). While the delivery of oral health services is not so simple, the same method can be applied. Once again, the additional service you offer or promote must be legally and ethically within your scope of practice and consistent with clients' needs. For example, many practices do not provide topical fluoride treatments for their adult patients, despite the fact that the efficacy of topical fluorides is well established. The usual justification for this is that insurance doesn't cover adult fluoride treatments. Insurance underwriters, however, are not in any position to make a professional judgment regarding the individual treatment needs of your clients. If it is within ethical bounds, and you add an additional $10 fluoride treatment to the maintenance visits of 75% of your adult patients (estimating that the remaining 25% either don't need or elect not to have fluoride), you will increase the income from a $30 maintenance visit by 30%.

Whether you choose to work toward increasing your average transaction price will depend on many factors, including professional ethics and clients' treatment needs, financial status, and expectations. For example, if most of your adult clients simply cannot afford to pay for fluoride treatments, you may lose a significant number of clients (and all associated income) by increasing the average transaction price. On the other hand, if these clients are badly in need of topical fluoride treatments, you have an ethical obligation to explain the necessity of this treatment. A decreased incidence of caries will save the clients money in the long run. Although this might decrease the practice income from restorative procedures, it might lead to increased referrals from satisfied clients.

Unfortunately, a well-known method of increasing the transaction price is to perform a simple procedure and bill for a similar, but more complex one. This practice is not only unethical, but illegal. Insurance companies and licensing boards are familiar with this scam, and no practice can get away with it indefinitely. Furthermore, healthcare consumers are becoming very sensitive to healthcare costs and are increasingly able to identify unscrupulous practices on their own. Loss of client goodwill, and clients, can be financially devastating. Increasing the average transaction price can be a successful method of increasing sales revenue, but only if everyone on the staff is sensitive to the ethical issues involved.

Some practices also increase sales revenue by selling oral healthcare products to their clients. The advantage is increased income without a significant increase in salary and personnel costs. If your existing staff can handle all the inventory, sales, and administrative functions, the only new cost you will incur is the cost of goods sold. The decision to go into product sales needs careful consideration and analysis. You must decide if product sales are consistent with the mission and goals of your practice. You must be sure that most of your clients are interested in purchasing oral health products from you. Some may appreciate the convenience and being able to make an informed decision with the help of a knowledgeable staff person. Others may be offended and consider in-office product sales "unprofessional." As with all marketing questions, you must learn what your clients want and provide that, not something more or something less. It may be difficult to make an objective decision on how your clients, or specific market niches, will respond to product sales. Approach the matter carefully, with sensitivity to all the feedback (both verbal and nonverbal). Increased revenue from product sales may, or may not, offset revenue lost if clients leave the practice.

"Selling" healthcare can be controversial. As healthcare reform continues, however, both practitioners and clients will be exploring new options. Practice managers should be sensitive to client interests.

## ADVERTISING

You may or may not choose to advertise your practice or services. The decision will be based on the mission, goals, and resources of your practice. Since the early seventies, the advertising of professional services has become more common. There are certainly many marketing activities, other than advertising, which you may choose to use in place of, or in conjunction with, advertising. Additionally, you may choose to advertise to only some of your clients (specific market segments) or to advertise only some of your services. Be aware that state licensing boards and professional ethics proscribe some strict practices for advertising professional services. For example, in most cases you cannot advertise that your services are "pain free" or that you offer specific drugs for pain control. Be sure that all those involved in ad development are aware of these restrictions and that each ad is reviewed by someone knowledgeable about the restrictions that apply to your field and your location. If you decide that advertising is consistent with the mission and image of your practice, there are a number media choices available.

Print media, usually the least expensive, include the phone book, newspapers, magazines, billboards, direct mail, and brochures/flyers. While most healthcare practices choose to have a listing in the yellow pages section of the phone book, not all choose to use a space ad. Metropolitan areas often have a proliferation of phone books, some for business only, some for the local area, some for the entire area. You will have to pay for each listing or ad. Plan your marketing strategy accordingly. You may choose to work with an advertising agency to design and place your ads if you will be going into newspapers and magazines, unless someone on the staff is knowledgeable about advertising. If you have adequate computer capability, you may be able to produce your own direct mail pieces or brochures in-house.

Other advertising media include radio and television. Although the production and placement of these ads can be costly, don't automatically rule them out of your advertising campaign. Local radio and cable TV station rates are often affordable; check to see whether the rates in your area are within your advertising budget. The cost per contact can be low because radio and TV can reach such large numbers of people. It is not the number of people reached that is important, but the number of people reached within your target audience. If your ad is seen or heard by 2 million people, and only 10 of them match your market profile (the group you are trying to reach), you have paid to advertise to 1,999,990 people whom your ad was not intended to interest.

Even if radio or TV is affordable, don't forget to consider whether or not a radio or TV ad will reach the right audience and be the right vehicle. As mentioned previously, don't overlook opportunities to do joint advertising with other healthcare providers, businesses, or community groups. Depending on the message, joint efforts may be more public relations activities than advertising, but whatever the case, the shared cost may be easier to bear. As with all your marketing activities, be sure that you are prepared to deal with the response to your ad. If your phone lines are completely tied up with calls responding to your ads, or clients suddenly have to wait three months for an appointment, you may be losing as many clients as you are gaining.

Be sure that each ad and placement is part of your overall marketing strategy and reaches a specific market segment with a specific message. Some messages, such as newspaper ads, reach a broad audience. You may only want to announce your availability, location, and phone number. Some messages can be more specific. For example, if the paper is running a section on cosmetic surgery, you may want to advertise your cosmetic dentistry services. If you offer a smoking cessation program, you may want to have a joint ad or campaign with the local heart association or physicians' group.

A vital part of any advertising campaign or ad placement is evaluation. If you plan to advertise, have mechanisms in place to track responses to your ads. This is usually as simple as asking "How did you find us?" or "Did you see our ad?" With this information, you will be able to evaluate the cost effectiveness of your ads. For example, if your yellow pages listing costs you $300 per year, and no one ever calls you as a result, something needs to change. Are you in the wrong book? Do you need an ad instead of just a listing? Do you need a different message? On the other hand, if your $300 listing brings in three new clients, it has been cost effective.

A more subjective evaluation is the quality of leads an ad brings in. Are your ads reaching the right audience? For example, if your newspaper ad is attracting new clients who cannot pay your fees, you will have to make adjustments. You can change the ad, place it elsewhere, lower your fees, or implement a new payment plan. You will have to decide whether this is a market segment you need to serve, either as a community service or because it is consistent with your strategic plan. Even your advertising mistakes can be enlightening. For example, you place an ad that is intended to attract retired persons to your practice and get many calls from the homebound requesting treatment. This may indicate that there is a market for a mobile service and may prompt you to plan and implement a new service.

Here are some examples of messages a dental, or dental hygiene, practice, might want to use. Even a dental practice that wholly controls its dental hygiene practice might want to promote its dental hygiene services specifically, as well as restorative or cosmetic services. Note that each message is tailored to fit the interests of a specific market segment.

If advertising in a support group newsletter to reach the physically challenged, state that your facilities are equipped for handicapped access. Although it is almost always a legal requirement that public facilities, such as dental offices, be handicapped accessible, this statement in your ad indicates your commitment to serving this group. Additionally, handicapped accessible doesn't necessarily mean easily accessible, and if your practice is more easily accessible than others, this is an important selling point. Your ad might also emphasize the need for regular preventive treatment and maintenance (e.g., dental hygiene) visits. The need for regular oral healthcare visits may be overlooked by individuals dealing with complex situations and your ad can serve as a reminder of the importance of maintaining good oral health. Additionally, your ad in the support group newsletter indicates a commitment to working with, and supporting, this community.

If advertising your cosmetic services in the beauty section of the local paper, include high quality (color, if possible) photographs in your ad. Be specific about the possible benefits of your cosmetic services, such as "remove coffee and tobacco stain," or "repair broken or damaged teeth." Before and after photos can say volumes about the effects of treatment. Other benefits for clients from cosmetic treatment may include more sales appeal with customers, or a more professional image. Cosmetic services lend themselves especially well to TV advertising.

In school or league sports programs, advertise that you make custom athletic mouth guards. Include a photo of a smiling local team member wearing one of your (almost undetectable) mouth guards. This ad will not only reach a specific audience but also deliver an important public health message and the ad revenue will support the local team. Public health messages, while not strictly advertising, often get good coverage on radio.

As with all other marketing activities, advertising ideas are limitless. Get ideas, and feedback, from staff, clients, and colleagues. Look at everyone else's ads, especially if you know they are successful. There may be many ideas that can be adapted to your practice.

## *Summary*

Marketing oral healthcare services is a creative endeavor with endless possibilities of activities. The process, however, is similar for all cases: Find a need and fill it. First, discover what oral healthcare services are needed in the communities you serve and find ways for your practice to fill those needs. Define your target markets, based on your research, and develop a marketing plan. If possible, pilot test your marketing activities, then implement and evaluate the activities. Refine and update your marketing continuously.

## *Review Questions*

1. State the importance of market research.
2. Describe a client database.
3. Describe marketing price, position, and promotion.
4. Describe the role of public relations in marketing oral healthcare delivery.
5. Describe some of the ethical considerations involved in "selling" healthcare.
6. Describe the role of advertising in marketing oral healthcare delivery.
7. Describe the process of marketing oral healthcare delivery.
8. Using a practice with which you are familiar (or a hypothetical one) as an example, describe the information you might collect in the client database.
9. Using a practice with which you are familiar (or a hypothetical one) as an example, describe its marketing position, pricing, and promotional activities.
10. Give an example of a public relations activity targeted at the
    a. community.
    b. clients.
    c. staff.
11. Describe three marketing activities targeting healthcare professionals.
12. You have a mobile dental hygiene practice. Describe one market niche for your services and marketing activities targeting that group.

13. You are the manager of a small dental practice in a suburban area and you want to promote your cosmetic dental services. Describe one market niche you want to reach. Describe how that group would benefit from your services. Describe marketing activities targeting them.

14. Working with an existing practice, develop a marketing plan for one of its service areas (i.e., hygiene, restorative, surgery). Your marketing plan should include a market analysis (information from the client database), a projection of market share increases resulting from the marketing activities, a description of the overall marketing plan, and descriptions of at least three marketing activities with cost estimates.

## SUGGESTED READING

Cooper, T. M., & Diabiaggio, J. A. (1979). *Applied practice management.* St. Louis: C.V. Mosby.

Haver, J. F., & Hanlon, M. A. (1983). *Personalized guide to marketing strategy.* Mosby's Dental Practice Management Series. St. Louis: C.V. Mosby.

Milone, C. L., Blair, W. C., & Littlefield, J. E. (1982). *Marketing for the dental practice.* Philadelphia: Saunders Publishing.

# CHAPTER 10

# Client Management

## Objectives

After reading this chapter and completing the review questions, the reader should be able to:

- List at least three rights that clients have in receiving oral healthcare.
- Explain one method of managing challenging children.
- Compare the use of 15-minute and 10-minute units in appointment scheduling.
- Discuss the advantages and disadvantages of leaving block time open in the schedule.
- State three reasons for establishing policies on missed appointments and late arrivals.
- List three factors to consider in establishing policy on missed appointments and late arrivals.
- Discuss two alternatives to charging for missed appointments.
- Discuss the advantages of confirming appointments.
- State the importance of good client management.
- Discuss the pros and cons of requiring payment at the time of service.
- Describe one method of doing case presentations.
- Discuss the pros and cons of office insurance processing.
- Discuss the three elements of a continuing care system.

The term *client* can refer to groups, businesses, or individuals and has been used throughout this text interchangeably with these terms. In this chapter, most of the discussion is related to the management of individual clients. Good client management is no more an accident than is good employee management. It requires thought, planning, skill, and ongoing evaluation. There are as many ways to approach client management as there are individual clients, and although you will need to make adjustments for each individual, it is important to have existing plans and policies in place. This will promote consistency in the approach used by all staff members and help prevent most client management problems from occurring.

## CLIENT RIGHTS

As has been mentioned in previous chapters, the relationships between your practice and staff and your clients have many associated legal implications. All staff members, including practice owners, need specific training in this area. Woodall and Bentley's text *Legal, Ethical and Management Aspects of the Dental Care System* (1983) is an excellent reference. Because legal issues may be subject to frequent and rapid change, it is advisable to have the entire staff participate in risk management training on a regular basis (every one or two years).

The rights of your clients must always be a primary consideration. Each, regardless of age or other considerations, deserves to be treated with respect, just as you would expect to be treated yourself. Woodall and Bentley offer a good summary of the relationship between practitioners and clients:

> It has been shown that when a patient seeks and accepts care from a health care provider, the patient enters a contractual relationship with the health care professional, and the health care professional is obligated to provide the care agreed to, according to the accepted standard of skill and care. The patient is expected to cooperate in the provision of care and to pay a reasonable fee for the services received.

The dentists and hygienists in a practice have a legal and ethical obligation to provide competent care for their clients and to be compensated (directly or indirectly) for their services. Clients have a right to be informed about their health and oral health status, to have treatment options and office policies (fees, billing, etc.) explained to them, and to make choices about the type of treatment they prefer. In other words, each client should be presented a treatment plan before treatment begins, even if it is a continuing care appointment with the dental hygienist. This does not need to be a long, involved case presentation, just a simple summary of the treatment planned for the visit. The most important factor in this process is that the client accepts the proposed treatment and agrees to the procedures to be performed.

For example, if the dentist tells the client that she will be putting a filling in a first molar and proceeds to fill the second molar at the same time, without informing the patient in advance, she has technically committed assault. It is irrelevant whether the second molar needed a restoration. This is especially true when treating minors. Providers must have the specific consent of the guardians for treatment procedures. Providers also have an ethical responsibility to inform minors, in language the client can understand, what procedures are to be performed.

For scheduling purposes, it is often convenient to book a block of time for restorative treatment for clients who have a variety of such needs (e.g., many amalgams). This works well for the practice because these appointments can remain flexible until the last minute, allowing for adaptation of the schedule to unexpected events, such as emergencies.

Each client record should contain a complete treatment plan, listing all the treatment the client needs. During the case presentation (formal or informal), the client agrees to some course of treatment and begins to schedule appointments as needed. It is fine to schedule a one- to two-hour restorative appointment, but at the start of the appointment, the dentist should outline the treatment to be performed at that visit and the client should agree to the plan. It is fine to agree that you will work on tooth number 2, and time permitting, number 3 as well. It is not a good idea to say you will work on the upper right and then do whatever time allows.

Children are at the mercy of adults. They should not be restrained or disciplined unless absolutely necessary, and never without the consent of a parent or guardian. If a child is combative or uncooperative, reschedule the appointment. Consult with the child's parent or guardian regarding behavioral problems and consider referral to a pediatric practice for treatment. Especially difficult or fearful children may need to be sedated to complete vitally necessary treatment. It is best to take as many short appointments as necessary to gain the child's (and parents') cooperation rather than to act hastily and violate the child's rights. It is better to lose a client than to permanently damage a child's self-esteem.

An excellent way to prepare the practice to handle challenging children is to establish good working relationships with pediatric practices in your area. Difficult cases can then be referred to them immediately, and you will reduce unpleasantness for both your clients and your staff and prevent children from developing life-long dental phobias. If you manage a pediatric practice, be prepared to accept the most challenging cases in your area. In fact, it can be an excellent marketing tool to promote these services. Your staff will need specific training in handling these cases and ongoing stress-reduction activities as well.

## APPOINTMENT SCHEDULING

One of the first decisions to be made regarding client management is appointment scheduling. The method you choose will depend on your staff resources (numbers of providers, administrative support, office technology, etc.). Evaluate your procedures from time to time. They may need modification.

Many types of appointment books, both manual and electronic, are available. Most schedules use set appointment units, usually in increments of 10 or 15 minutes. The unit length determines the times listed on the appointment schedule. For example, using 10-minute units, an appointment schedule from 9 A.M. to 10 A.M. would list appointment times for 9:00, 9:10, 9:20, 9:30, 9:40, 9:50, and 10:00.

Using 15-minute units, an appointment schedule from 9 A.M. to 10 A.M. would list appointment times for 9:00, 9:15, 9:30, 9:45, and 10:00. There can be advantages to both systems, but 10-minute units usually allow more flexibility in the schedule and promote efficient use of provider time.

Figures 10.1 through 10.6 are examples of various appointment schedules. Figure 10.1 is the simplest. It is the schedule for a solo dental practice in which there is one dentist and one assistant, working out of one treatment room. Even if this practice were using two treatment rooms, they might continue with this same schedule. An alternative would be to use two columns in the appointment book, one for each treatment room (as in Figure 10.5) so that overlapping appointments would be clear in the schedule. Booking overlapping appointments is useful for appointments that do not require all of the provider's time continuously.

Regardless of the number of providers, assistants, or available treatment rooms, it is *inadvisable* to leave clients alone in treatment rooms. Clients may be anxious about dental procedures and need reassurance. Clients may expect personal service and will not appreciate being "ignored." No client who has received any medication in your office, including local anesthesia, should ever be left alone, in case the client experiences a reaction to the medication. The same precaution should be followed for every client who has any foreign objects in the mouth, such as cotton rolls, rubber dams, impression materials, or uncemented appliances (crowns, etc.) in case the client chokes or aspirates the material. If you never leave clients alone in the treatment rooms, this should also reduce theft. Finally, it should be common courtesy to have a staff member keep clients company. This provides a perfect opportunity for informal conversation. You will gain valuable information about client interests and suggestions for your practice.

Figure 10.2 is a schedule using 10-minute units for a practice with one dentist, one hygienist, and three treatment rooms. This schedule uses two columns, one for each provider. The third treatment room is available to both providers, to use as needed, but is not specifically assigned for particular use on the schedule. Notice that in both the dentist's and hygienist's schedules, clients are not appointed for fixed-length appointments, but rather for variable-length appointments as needed.

Figures 10.3 and 10.4 are schedules for dental hygienists. Compare the two and notice the increased productivity achieved using 10-minute units. The hygienist in Figure 10.3 treats six adults and two children, whereas the hygienist in Figure 10.4 treats six adults and four children. Productivity was increased by giving the adult patients variable-length appointments, based on their treatment needs.

Figure 10.5 is a dentist's schedule. The dentist works in two treatment rooms with one assistant. Scheduling forms are available that indicate both the dentist's time and the assistant's time. Although scheduling both these times requires some special training and extra work for the receptionist, it may increase provider productivity. Notice the increased productivity for the dentist, as compared to Figure 10.1. The major difference is the second treatment room, but 10-minute units and increased function of the assistant are important factors as well. Notice that blocks of time are left open before lunch and at the end of the day to treat emergencies.

Figure 10.6 is the schedule of an accelerated dental hygiene practice. The dentist's schedule is not shown; his exam time is included within the client's block of time. The dental hygienist works out of two treatment rooms with one assistant. Because most clients are given one-hour appointments, a schedule using 15-minute units might also provide sufficient detail. More information on accelerated dental hygiene practice is given in Chapter 6.

| | |
|---|---|
| 9:00 | Mr. Longhurst |
| 9:15 | MOD #30 |
| 9:30 | |
| 9:45 | ▼ |
| 10:00 | Ben Grant |
| 10:15 | maintenance |
| 10:30 | ▼ |
| 10:45 | Robin Todd |
| 11:00 | crown prep 2–4 |
| 11:15 | |
| 11:30 | |
| 11:45 | ▼ |
| 12:00 | lunch |
| 12:15 | |
| 12:30 | |
| 12:45 | ▼ |
| 1:00 | Alice Burns |
| 1:15 | new patient |
| 1:30 | |
| 1:45 | |
| 2:00 | ▼ |
| 2:15 | Ms. Adams |
| 2:30 | ▼ adj. denture |
| 2:45 | Wendell Rover |
| 3:00 | restorative |
| 3:15 | ▼ |
| 3:30 | |
| 3:45 | Mr. Taylor |
| 4:00 | maintenance |
| 4:15 | ▼ |
| 4:30 | W. Tucker |
| 4:45 | ▼ seat crown #4 |
| 5:00 | |

*Note:* A real schedule would include phone numbers and notations of appointment confirmation.

**Figure 10.1**   *Solo practice, 15-minute units*

| | Dr. Jones | Ms. Smith |
|---|---|---|
| 9:00 | S. Dickerson | B. Tribble |
| 9:10 | ▼ adj. #18 | maintenance |
| 9:20 | Allen Hammond | |
| 9:30 | new patient | |
| 9:40 | ▼ | ▼ |
| 9:50 | Brooke Gregory | M. Alonzo |
| 10:00 | restorative | new patient |
| 10:10 | | |
| 10:20 | | |
| 10:30 | | |
| 10:40 | S. Briggs | ▼ |
| 10:50 | ▼ consult | |
| 11:00 | M. Alonzo | Norman Rose |
| 11:10 | ▼ exam, tx. plan | scale/rt. plane |
| 11:20 | J. Field | |
| 11:30 | ext. #15 | |
| 11:40 | | |
| 11:50 | ▼ | ▼ |
| 12:00 | lunch | lunch |
| 12:10 | | |
| 12:20 | | |
| 12:30 | | |
| 12:40 | | |
| 12:50 | ▼ | ▼ |
| 1:00 | M. Thomas | H. Lovell |
| 1:10 | bridge prep | maintenance |
| 1:20 | | |
| 1:30 | | ▼ |
| 1:40 | | Sally Harper |
| 1:50 | ▼ | maintenance |
| 2:00 | Debra Sewell | |
| 2:10 | bond 7–10 | |
| 2:20 | | ▼ |
| 2:30 | | Faith Allen |
| 2:40 | | sealants |
| 2:50 | ▼ | ▼ |
| 3:00 | Ms. Brown | Jessica Brown |
| 3:10 | restorative | maintenance |
| 3:20 | | ▼ |
| 3:30 | ▼ | Tommy Brown |
| 3:40 | Ms. Sellars | maintenance |
| 3:50 | pain ULQ | |
| 4:00 | ▼ | H. Yates |
| 4:10 | Avery Williams | new patient |
| 4:20 | rest. #2 and 3 | |
| 4:30 | | |
| 4:40 | ▼ | |
| 4:50 | Dan Willcox | |
| 5:00 | ▼ impression | ▼ |

*Note:* A real schedule would include phone numbers and notations of appointment confirmation.

**Figure 10.2**    *One dentist, one hygienist, 10-minute units*

|  |  |
|------|-------------|
| 9:00 | Bill Hanson |
| 9:15 | maintenance |
| 9:30 | |
| 9:45 | Arthur Blum |
| 10:00 | maintenance |
| 10:15 | |
| 10:30 | Choa Hung |
| 10:45 | scale/rt. plane |
| 11:00 | |
| 11:15 | |
| 11:30 | |
| 11:45 | |
| 12:00 | lunch |
| 12:15 | |
| 12:30 | |
| 12:45 | |
| 1:00 | Rick Hunt |
| 1:15 | scale/rt. plane |
| 1:30 | |
| 1:45 | |
| 2:00 | |
| 2:15 | |
| 2:30 | Mr. Perry |
| 2:45 | re-check |
| 3:00 | Trevor Perry |
| 3:15 | maintenance |
| 3:30 | Kevin Donalson |
| 3:45 | sealants |
| 4:00 | Wes Hall |
| 4:15 | new patient |
| 4:30 | |
| 4:45 | |
| 5:00 | |

*Note:* A real schedule would include phone numbers and notations of appointment confirmation.

**Figure 10.3**   *Hygienist, 15-minute units*

|  | | |
|------|------|------|
| 9:00 | Gary Pecore | |
| 9:10 | | maintenance |
| 9:20 | | |
| 9:30 | | |
| 9:40 | | |
| 9:50 | | ↓ |
| 10:00 | CJ Schmidt | |
| 10:10 | | maintenance |
| 10:20 | | |
| 10:30 | | ↓ |
| 10:40 | Peg Hanston | |
| 10:50 | | maintenance |
| 11:00 | | |
| 11:10 | | |
| 11:20 | | ↓ |
| 11:30 | Barbara Buck | |
| 11:40 | | scale/rt. plane |
| 11:50 | | |
| 12:00 | lunch | |
| 12:10 | | |
| 12:20 | | |
| 12:30 | | |
| 12:40 | | |
| 12:50 | | ↓ |
| 1:00 | James Hack | |
| 1:10 | | OHI and micro |
| 1:20 | | |
| 1:30 | | ↓ |
| 1:40 | Jon Tracy | |
| 1:50 | | maintenance |
| 2:00 | | ↓ |
| 2:10 | Julie Peck | |
| 2:20 | | maintenance |
| 2:30 | | ↓ |
| 2:40 | Joel Peck | |
| 2:50 | | sealants |
| 3:00 | | |
| 3:10 | | ↓ |
| 3:20 | Allison Scanlon | |
| 3:30 | | maintenance |
| 3:40 | | ↓ |
| 3:50 | Collin Trager | |
| 4:00 | | new patient |
| 4:10 | | |
| 4:20 | | |
| 4:30 | | |
| 4:40 | | |
| 4:50 | | ↓ |
| 5:00 | | |

*Note:* A real schedule would include phone numbers and notations of appointment confirmation.

**Figure 10.4**    *Hygienist, 10-minute units*

| | Room 1 | Room 2 |
|---|---|---|
| 9:00 | George Dargan | Eve Danoff |
| 9:10 | rest #12 | adj. #18 |
| 9:20 | | ▼ |
| 9:30 | ▼ | Mr. Tindal |
| 9:40 | | crown prep #2 & 3 |
| 9:50 | | |
| 10:00 | | |
| 10:10 | | ▼ |
| 10:20 | Dale Lawne | |
| 10:30 | RCT #6 | |
| 10:40 | | |
| 10:50 | | |
| 11:00 | | |
| 11:10 | ▼ | B. Sheldon |
| 11:20 | | ▼ impressions |
| 11:30 | emergency | emergency |
| 11:40 | | |
| 11:50 | | ▼ |
| 12:00 | lunch | lunch |
| 12:10 | | |
| 12:20 | | |
| 12:30 | | |
| 12:40 | | |
| 12:50 | ▼ | ▼ |
| 1:00 | Brian Sharp | |
| 1:10 | seat crown | |
| 1:20 | | Charles McGee |
| 1:30 | ▼ | new patient |
| 1:40 | | |
| 1:50 | | |
| 2:00 | | |
| 2:10 | Joe Huff | |
| 2:20 | restorative | |
| 2:30 | | ▼ |
| 2:40 | | Chris Bowlen |
| 2:50 | | restorative |
| 3:00 | | ▼ |
| 3:10 | Ms. Seiling | |
| 3:20 | ext. #14 & 15 | |
| 3:30 | | |
| 3:40 | | |
| 3:50 | ▼ | |
| 4:00 | Shannon Smith | |
| 4:10 | consult | Ken Montgomery |
| 4:20 | | start bridge #18-20 |
| 4:30 | | |
| 4:40 | | |
| 4:50 | ▼ | ▼ |
| 5:00 | | |

*Note:* A real schedule would include phone numbers and notations of appointment confirmation.

**Figure 10.5** *One dentist, two rooms*

|  | Room A | Room B |
|---|---|---|
| 9:00 | K. Pfeifer | |
| 9:10 | maintenance | |
| 9:20 | | |
| 9:30 | | John Dobbin |
| 9:40 | | maintenance |
| 9:50 | ↓ | |
| 10:00 | Tom Bryne | |
| 10:10 | 1 qd. SC/RP | |
| 10:20 | | ↓ |
| 10:30 | | Katherine Dorsey |
| 10:40 | | maintenance |
| 10:50 | ↓ | |
| 11:00 | Mr. McCarthy | |
| 11:10 | maintenance | |
| 11:20 | | ↓ |
| 11:30 | | Mr. Bartholow |
| 11:40 | | re-check |
| 11:50 | ↓ | ↓ |
| 12:00 | lunch | lunch |
| 12:10 | | |
| 12:20 | | |
| 12:30 | | |
| 12:40 | | |
| 12:50 | ↓ | ↓ |
| 1:00 | AF Cohen | |
| 1:10 | maintenance | |
| 1:20 | | |
| 1:30 | | Scott Baron |
| 1:40 | | 1 qd. SC/RP |
| 1:50 | ↓ | |
| 2:00 | Mike Patel | |
| 2:10 | maintenance | |
| 2:20 | | ↓ |
| 2:30 | | Matt Malone |
| 2:40 | | maintenance |
| 2:50 | ↓ | ↓ |
| 3:00 | Jed Cleveland | Justin Cleveland |
| 3:10 | maintenance | maintenance |
| 3:20 | ↓ | ↓ |
| 3:30 | Sandy Payne | Andy Jones |
| 3:40 | maintenance | maintenance |
| 3:50 | ↓ | |
| 4:00 | Nick Brown | |
| 4:10 | sealants | |
| 4:20 | | ↓ |
| 4:30 | | Jimmy Ubel |
| 4:40 | | maintenance |
| 4:50 | ↓ | ↓ |
| 5:00 | | |

*Note:* A real schedule would include phone numbers and notations of appointment confirmation.

**Figure 10.6**   *Accelerated DHPC*

## Scheduling Problems

Many factors should be taken into consideration in planning the appointment schedule, including treating emergencies (this usually applies only to dental practice) and the use of block time. Emergencies will occur. Plan how you will deal with them. One method is to leave time open each day (as in Figure 10.5) to use for emergencies or as a buffer, to allow for running over time with other appointments. If you work emergencies into the schedule, either with or without open time, consider how the bulk of your clients will react to waiting. You will know if the waiting time is a problem for clients because they will either complain or stop seeing you. Don't ignore these symptoms.

Staff stress is another effect of overscheduling, affecting providers and staff members, especially if this is a chronic occurrence. Beyond the demands of producing good work without adequate time, you will all have disgruntled clients to deal with. If overscheduling or running behind schedule is causing problems, deal with them. If this is to be a fact of work life in your practice, incorporate stress-reduction activities.

Client management can have a significant impact on scheduling problems. Clients who are habitually late or miss appointments are the chief culprits. You must establish a firm policy regarding late and missed appointments and apply it consistently. The policy you create will be determined by your clients, staff, and resources. Although you are generally trying to customize your service to appeal specifically to the various market niches that you serve, it is important that your scheduling procedures, especially concerning late or missed appointments, be applicable to most of your clients. You cannot allow one small group of clients to throw the entire office schedule into chaos. Additionally, staff members must be able to cope with scheduling policies and remain productive. You must make the scheduling policies clear during the hiring process so that you are bringing on staff members who can work within your system. Other resources to consider in establishing scheduling policies are space in the reception area and number of treatment rooms. If waiting clients and overlapping appointments are part of your plan, be sure that you have the physical space to accommodate them.

Establish a policy for clients arriving late for their appointments. What time interval is unacceptable? At what point will you refuse to see them (they will have to be reappointed)? Ten minutes is probably a minimum. The maximum will depend on factors mentioned earlier. To manage your clients, make this policy clear. Have the receptionist explain to clients that if they are more than, for example, 10 minutes late, they will have to make another appointment and that this policy assures that all clients are treated fairly and are not kept waiting.

Clients arriving on time deserve to be treated on time. Even clients who are reappointed will appreciate this policy when they arrive on time and are not kept waiting for someone else who arrives late. Note that this implies a commitment on your part. If you cannot wait more than 10 minutes (or whatever interval you choose) for your clients, they should not wait more than 10 minutes for you. This will involve close work with providers and assistants to ensure that they can handle their schedules. If some staff members have problems, either modify your policies or change staff. If the problem providers are practice owners, they will have to understand the impact their tardiness is having on clients, staff, and office policies. Staff meetings and strategic planning sessions are good times to address these issues as a group. Individual problems should be handled individually.

If your late policy causes you to lose clients, you will have to evaluate the variables involved. If you are losing only a few clients, you are only eliminating those who would have upset the entire schedule and angered all your other clients. On the other hand, if your late policy is causing many clients to leave, you will have to modify your policy (or give up that part of your market). Additionally, someone has to have the authority to make exceptions to this policy. Clearly establish, in advance, who will have this authority. Do not discuss these exceptions in the reception area in front of other clients. Do this in a private office.

Establish your policy on missed appointments in a similar manner. Decide what the policy will be based on clients, staff, and resources—and apply it consistently. Clearly establish who has the authority to make exceptions and do this privately. Make adjustments based on market demand. Missed appointments greatly decrease production and practice revenues and so must be held to a minimum.

If you are a fee-for-service practice (not a free clinic), you should charge for missed appointments after a minimum number of infractions. Be generous with the minimum. You don't have to tell clients what it is. Usually just stating the policy of charging for missed appointments is sufficient to remind clients of their commitments to you. The charge for missed appointments should be in line with your other fees. It should be high enough to be noticed, but not unreasonable. The charge for a missed appointment should not be higher than the treatment fees. Usually one or two charges for missed appointments will persuade problem clients to keep their appointments or to go elsewhere for treatment.

Some clients will never be reliable about keeping appointments. This is especially true of those receiving free treatment. You certainly can't charge them for missed appointments, and most public health facilities cannot refuse to treat individuals who qualify for their services, even if these individuals miss most of their appointments. If your clients chronically miss appointments, you will have to adjust your scheduling policies accordingly. You can do this by double or triple booking or by accepting low productivity. If half or more of your clients miss their appointments, you can safely double book, although this may cause some staff stress if two clients do show up at the same time. Certainly, if you have this many clients missing appointments, you can ask them to wait. Another option is to explain that something has come up, either an emergency or staff shortage, and ask one of the clients to reschedule. If the staff has trouble adjusting to double booking, low productivity may be an option, depending on the mission of your practice. If you have low productivity due to missed appointments, you can partially offset the lost revenue by reducing staff size and other space and equipment costs. If you are seeing fewer clients, you should be able to get by with fewer resources.

## Confirming Appointments

Regardless of your practice setting and mission, clients get busy and not everyone is good at time management. It is important that your clients come in for their appointments and come in on time. The cost of confirming appointments is much lower than the cost of missed or unfilled appointments. Phone to confirm all appointments about 24 hours in advance. Confirming appointments may be the responsibility of one person, or may be a task shared by several during their downtime from clinical duties. Remember that these confirmation calls are contacts with your clients and should therefore be part of your marketing and quality assurance programs. Anyone handling these client calls (or others) should have training. Many community colleges, professional groups, and private companies offer training in customer service and, specifically, handling telephone calls. The cost of good training is a worthwhile investment. A few clients lost due to lack of staff communication skills can be costly.

When calling to confirm appointments, be sure to mention all necessary information, including the name and phone number of the practice, name of the person calling, and the time and length of the client's appointment. Also mention which provider the appointment is with, the treatment planned, and any specific instructions for the client, such as taking antibiotic premedication. Mention any other information specific to your practice, such as parking arrangements. If it is necessary to leave a message to confirm an appointment, remember that health and treatment information is confidential. It is helpful to inform the client at the time an appointment is made and at the time of confirmation how long the appointment will last, not just the start time, so that clients understand how long you have set aside for them. If there is more than one provider in your practice, clients need to be reminded who they will be seeing and why. This prevents misunderstandings. The client knows in advance who will be treating him and what will be done.

New clients should be reminded to come at least 15 minutes early to complete necessary paperwork, especially health history information. Remind them that this information will be collected and to be prepared with the names of their physicians and previous dentist(s), names and doses of their present medications, insurance and any other information you need them to bring.

If, at the time of confirmation, a client mentions that he may be late, remind him of the office policy regarding lateness or appointments canceled with less than 24 hours' notice. Accommodate the client as much as possible, but apply office policies consistently and politely.

Regardless of the market you serve, the best approach to client management is good client relations. Keep your commitments to your clients and they will be more inclined to keep their commitments to you. Demonstrate that you care about their well-being and the quality of services you provide; work with them as though they were partners in your practice. Most people will respond to this type of involvement and eliminate your client management problems for you.

## COMMUNICATIONS

Every interaction that anyone in the practice has with any client is a marketing contact and should be handled accordingly. This implies that all staff members, including practice owners, must have adequate training to manage these interactions successfully. More information on marketing is contained in other chapters. This section deals with client management through good communications.

All of your client communications should be designed with the client in mind. Make it easy for clients to do business with you. Do not design your office, handouts, mailings, forms, and so on for ease of staff use. Your staff is being paid for their time. Your clients are not. Also, don't assume that the pieces that worked well 10 years ago are still the best ones to use. The environment, your clients, your staff, and many other factors change. Modify and update your client communications on a regular basis. These include your phone contacts and all written pieces, including billing and insurance forms. Your treatment forms and charts are not intended for client use and may be designed with staff convenience in mind. Your clients will, however, see their charts and forms and may request copies. Be sure that these are professional, neat, and in keeping with your practice image.

## Billing and Insurance Policies

Office policies, and forms for billing and insurance processing, are critical elements in client management. As with other office policies for clients, establish your billing policies based on client needs, staff input, and available resources. Apply your policies consistently, and establish clear lines of communication regarding exceptions. Evaluate your policies regularly and modify them as needed.

Make your billing and insurance policies clear to clients to prevent misunderstanding. Be sure that your bills are easy to read and understand, that the amount due is clearly stated and stands out, and that the due date is included. If you are collecting payment at the time of service, be sure that clients know this in advance, especially new clients. If you do bill, it is helpful to give clients a walk-out statement at the end of each visit, not only to provide them with a summary of their treatment for the day, but also to provide them with an opportunity to ask billing questions in person. You can clear up misunderstandings quickly, without letting resentment build up, and settle disputes quickly and directly.

There are pros and cons to asking for payment at the time of service. It certainly improves the cash flow of the practice and cuts down on billing costs. The downside is that many clients resent it, especially if they are asked to pay before treatment. Base your policies on the clients you serve. Some will be happy to pay in advance of or immediately following treatment if it reduces their costs. Some will be willing to pay a little more for the convenience and respect of being billed. As with scheduling policy, you will have to make billing policies that suit most of your patients, or you will not be able to apply them consistently.

There are exceptions, but asking for payment before delivering any service is a questionable marketing practice. People expect to get something for their money. If you ask them for money in advance, you are giving the message that your convenience is more important than theirs or that you do not trust them to pay you (which may be the case). This does not inspire client commitment to you or build loyalty—two factors that can be invaluable to your practice. If you must reduce collection time, it is far better to wait until the end of the appointment, after treatment, before asking for payment. As already mentioned, there can be many advantages to using walk-out statements, even if you do not ask for immediate payment.

Other billing policies to establish include finance charges on unpaid balances, payment for procedures requiring multiple visits and/or laboratory charges (i.e., crown and bridge), and payment plans for total case fees (i.e., orthodontics or total reconstruction). It is certainly reasonable to apply finance charges to unpaid balances, since they do cost the practice money. The finance charge rate, however, should be reasonable, for you are not in the banking business but are allowing the unpaid balance as a service to your clients. Finance charges should also be built into payment plans.

Communicating these financial issues to clients is important. Most people regard their finances as confidential, so you should make an effort to discuss billing matters privately, especially when discussing unpaid balances, finance charges, case fees, and late payments. These issues are also related to case presentations.

## Case Presentations

Clients deserve to have their conditions and treatment options clearly explained to them. It may be a dentist, hygienist, assistant, manager, or administrator who does formal case presentations, but dentists and hygienists need to provide their clients with health and treatment information. With new clients, and especially with clients presenting with a complicated case, it is a good idea to set time aside specifically for a case presentation. This should be done privately, with the client positioned in an up-right, face-to-face position. Providers should not be talking to the back of the client's head while he is reclined in the treatment chair.

The person doing the case presentation should have specific training in this area, regardless of his background. Information presented should include the client's present health and oral health status, all diagnostic tests and records (such as photographs, radiographs, models, charting), treatment options, associated costs, insurance information, and payment options. If the person presenting the case is not the one who prepared the diagnosis and treatment plan, it is important that the presenter understand this fully and that the healthcare provider be available to answer questions.

Depending on the resources of the practice, case presentations may be made in the treatment room, provided that this is not done during treatment and that the client is upright and facing the presenter. Practices charging premium fees or doing complex cases (such as orthodontics) should use a private office or consultation room for case presentations. Regardless of the setting, the client should be given a summary of the case presentation, including the agreed-upon treatment plan and payment plan. Maintain a copy of this record, either in the client's clinical file or in the business record. If the presentation summary is not in the client's file, be sure that there are notes in the clinical file regarding the treatment plan that the client has agreed upon. This is an important step in risk management.

Clients will call upon your office for all sorts of insurance information, much of which is only available through their insurance carrier or administrator. Regardless, they will expect you to be of service. There are two approaches you may take with insurance processing. The simplest one is to provide clients with a superbill or general-purpose computer-generated insurance form for each service rendered, perhaps in conjunction with a walk-out statement. The advantage to using this system, especially if the forms are generated by the office computer system, is that the form is generated at the conclusion of the visit. No separate claims processing is required, greatly reducing the amount of staff time spent processing insurance claims (which can be significant and costly). Clients then append the superbill or similar form to the insurance form and file the claim themselves. Clients are responsible to your office for all their charges and keep the reimbursement they receive from their insurance companies.

The disadvantage to this system is that many clients, even those with Ph.D.s, can't complete the claims process and are therefore never paid by their insurance companies. Their oral healthcare then becomes prohibitively expensive, and they start avoiding your practice. Additionally, many insurance carriers are starting to require that claims be processed electronically, a change that is incompatible with the client filing system. These types of problems can further delay or prevent your receiving payment for your services. For these reasons, many practices choose to file insurance claims for their clients.

If your practice will be submitting claims, you may still be able to use the superbill or computer-generated generic forms in most cases. The clients can assign their benefits to you, so that the practice receives the payment directly from the insurance company. This system requires that you have someone on staff well versed in claims processing and intimately familiar with the carriers in your area. Additionally, this will give you better understanding of the insurance pretreatment authorization process, which will enable you to help your clients with their treatment planning. The advantage to processing claims is that you will have more direct control of the communications with the insurance companies, will be better able to make claims effectively, and should receive payment in a more timely fashion. Many clients will rely on you for this type of service, although it can be costly to the practice. Further implications regarding billing, collections, and claims processing are discussed in Chapter 8.

## CONTINUING CARE

The continuing care process has been called many things, typically *recall,* also *maintenance,* sometimes *recare,* and others. While recall is probably the most common term, it has fallen into disfavor. Recall is something done for defective automobiles and appliances. From a marketing standpoint, it is best not to associate your practice with defects. The term you choose to use should reflect the value that you (and, hopefully) your clients place on their continuing health maintenance and care in your practice. What you call this program is less important than having an effective program in place.

The continuing care program is vital to dental hygiene practice, general dental practice, and periodontal practice. Other specialties should not lose touch with their existing clients, especially those in orthodontic treatment, but their continuing care or contact programs will differ from the three areas already mentioned, whose clients need to continue seeing them on a regular basis. You have an obligation to encourage your clients to maintain good health, and to remind them to visit you regularly is an important part of this process. The continuing care program is an important marketing tool as well.

The goal of a continuing care system is to maintain your active clients in your practice, for their health benefits and for your practice income. The continuing care program should include activities for making maintenance appointments, reminding clients that they are due for a visit, and purging inactive files.

You may choose to use many elements in your continuing care system, depending on your practice's resources and client interests. The continuing care program is vital to marketing the practice and the one element that keeps your clients with you. Attracting new clients is more difficult than keeping existing clients.

Some practices make maintenance appointments in advance, at the time of each maintenance visit. For example, clients coming in for recare in September on six-month maintenance would schedule an appointment for March at the conclusion of the September visit. The advantage is that clients have made a commitment to return to your practice and have their choice of appointment times. The disadvantage is that the appointment schedule fills up far ahead of time, making it more difficult for new clients to get appointments or for others to make necessary changes. If you do make appointments in advance, you will need a system for reminding clients of their appointments.

Two common reminder methods are postcards and phone calls. When using postcard reminders, clients address a reminder card to themselves when they schedule the visit. In this way, they are much more likely to notice and read a piece in their own handwriting. Alternatively you can use computer-generated labels or hand write the labels if this method is successful for you. The postcards are then filed by month and mailed to clients about a month before they are due for their appointments. The postcard system can also be used without making advance appointments. In this case, the cards are a reminder, not of a specific appointment the client has made, but to call you for an appointment.

Phone calls can also be used as reminders in the continuing care system. If you are appointing in advance, you call clients two to three weeks before their appointments to remind them of the appointments they made. You can also call to remind clients that it is time for a maintenance visit, even if you do not appoint them in advance. Phone calls can be used in conjunction with postcards. The reminder calls are not the same as confirmation calls. It is still a good idea to call clients 24 to 48 hours before each appointment to confirm that they are planning to come in. Some clients will appreciate all these phone calls and some will not. Some combination of all three methods (advance appointments, postcards, and phone calls) may work best, and you may choose to use different combinations for different clients.

One of the purposes of a continuing care system is to keep clients current. Part of the system should include purging inactive files. You will need to make a policy decision regarding what constitutes an active client. Is it someone who has been in for anything in the past three years? Someone who has been in for maintenance in the past two years? What efforts need to be made to contact clients before placing them on inactive status? Before placing clients on inactive status, make a final effort to contact them. Make notes in the charts regarding not only the date of inactivation, but the reason. This is important marketing data, but is also important for risk management. It should be clear in the chart that the client was not abandoned and that efforts were made to continue care.

To produce meaningful marketing plans, you need to have an accurate count of your active clients. Keeping this tally can be part of the continuing care system, or all of these may be functions that are part of your office computer system. A practice with fewer than about 2000 active clients can probably use a manual system effectively. Larger practices will probably need a computer for efficient operations. It is important that, manual or electronic, the system be orderly and kept up to date. No amount of technology can produce order out of chaos.

Waiting lists are related to the continuing care system. You may choose to have the receptionist keep a list of clients willing to come in on short notice or who want a specific appointment time, if one becomes available (usually Saturdays and evenings). Using the waiting list accommodates your clients' requests and is a critical element in maintaining productivity, because unfilled appointments greatly reduce provider productivity. The waiting list may not fill all the unfilled appointments, but it will help. Furthermore, each client record should include an up-to-date treatment plan, so that it is easy for all staff members to identify unfilled treatment needs—to remind clients (for health and marketing purposes) and to refer to when clients call with questions.

Maintaining the continuing care system should be a part of daily operations. It is a key element in practice success, especially dental hygiene practice. The system will work most effectively if it is an integral part of operations, and not just something hygienists do in their spare time. The clients in the continuing care system generate income not only for the DHPC but for dentistry as well. It is during maintenance visits that clients' dental treatment needs are most often identified. Clients who wait until something breaks or hurts to visit you are already unhappy when they walk in the door. It will be better for the practice and for clients to come in regularly, not just for emergencies.

## Summary

When establishing policies for client management, base your decisions on your clients, staff, and available resources. You need policies regarding scheduling, late arrivals and missed appointments, billing and insurance processing, plus any other client issues that occur in your practice. Apply the policies consistently. Clearly establish who has the authority to make exceptions, and do this privately. Review your policies frequently, and make adjustments based on market demand.

Regardless of the market you serve, the best approach to client management is good client relations. Keep your commitments to your clients, and they will keep their commitments to you. Demonstrate that you care about their well-being and the quality of services you provide; work with them as though they were partners in

your practice. Most people will respond positively and client management problems won't occur.

## Review Questions

1.  List at least three rights that clients have in receiving oral healthcare.
2.  Write a client bill of rights for a practice in which you are involved or for your
    ideal practice.
3.  Explain one method of managing challenging children.
4.  Compare the use of 15-minute and 10-minute units in appointment scheduling.
5.  Create an example appointment schedule. Explain your choices regarding
    time units and other scheduling policies. You may use an office you work in as
    part of the example, explaining which of its policies work best and which
    could be improved.
6.  Discuss the advantages and disadvantages of leaving block time open in the
    schedule.
7.  If you have ever worked in any healthcare practice that uses open block time,
    describe whether the system worked well there. Why or why not?
8.  State three reasons for establishing policies on missed appointments and late
    arrivals.
9.  List three factors to consider in establishing policy on missed appointments
    and late arrivals.
10. Discuss two alternatives to charging for missed appointments.
11. Using a practice with which you are familiar as an example, discuss the pros
    and cons of its policies on missed appointments and late arrivals.
12. Discuss the advantages of confirming appointments.
13. State the importance of good client management.
14. Discuss the pros and cons of requiring payment at the time of service.
15. Describe one method of doing case presentations.
16. Discuss the pros and cons of office insurance processing.
17. Discuss the three elements of a continuing care system.
18. Design a continuing care system for a practice with which you are familiar or
    for a hypothetical one. State your rationale for your choices.

## SUGGESTED READING

Finkbeiner, P. (1991). *Office procedures for the dental team* (3rd ed.). St. Louis: C.V. Mosby.

Treacy, M., & Wiersema, F. (1993). Customer intimacy and other value disciplines. *Harvard Business Review*, 71(1), 84–93.

Woodall, I., & Wiles, C. C. (1993). Formulating a treatment plan, case presentation and appointment plan. In *Comprehensive dental hygiene care* (4th ed.), edited by I. Woodall. St. Louis: C.V. Mosby.

## REFERENCES

Woodall, I., & Bentley, J. M. (1983). *Legal, ethical and management aspects of the dental care system* (2nd ed.). St. Louis: C.V. Mosby.

# PART 3

# THE DENTAL HYGIENIST AS MANAGER IN OTHER SETTINGS

*All types of businesses have managers, and managers come from many different backgrounds. Dental hygienist–managers are not limited to clinical practice. They can be found in many types of businesses.*

*Part 3 gives an overview of dental hygienists in four different management positions: education, product manufacturing, public health, and research. Each chapter has been written by a dental hygienist with management experience in a particular area and includes "how to" guidelines as well as discussion of each author's management experience and career development. These chapters are not intended to cover all there is to know about management in these types of businesses, but to tell the story of how these individuals, starting with a basic dental hygiene education, evolved into management roles.*

*Management roles for dental hygienists are not limited to these four areas. Hygienists are managing various other businesses, and new opportunities are created all the time by enterprising dental hygienists. This last part of the book is not intended to be a summary of the possibilities, but a springboard for generating new ideas.*

# CHAPTER 11

# Dental Hygiene Education

---

## Objectives

After reading this chapter and completing the review questions, the reader should be able to:

- List the seven functions for which the director of an academic program is responsible.
- Define what a dental hygiene program's commitment should be to teaching, research, and service.
- Define the director's role in the recruitment and development of program faculty.
- List the components of student personnel services.
- State the importance of the yearly budgetary process.
- Describe the evaluation processes that a dental hygiene program must go through.

---

## EDUCATIONAL LEADERSHIP

Providing leadership to the dental hygiene program in a college or university is the most vital function of the director. The success of the program, the quality of graduates, the ease with which the various groups cooperate, are related to the degree and the quality of educational leadership exercised by the director. It is the purpose of this chapter to discuss broad concepts of educational leadership in the administration of a collegiate dental hygiene program.

The administrative heads of dental hygiene programs have traditionally been called directors, although a few programs use the title *dean*. There are over 200 accredited dental hygiene programs, the majority of which (about 70%) are located in community colleges.

It is important to realize that in administering a dental hygiene program, both external and internal forces influence the program. One of the internal forces that needs to be taken into consideration is that dental hygiene education is a relatively new discipline in institutions of higher education. Interpretation of the objectives of the dental hygiene program to central administration, to chairs of other departments in the college, to faculty, and to students is important. The degree of understanding fostered by the dental hygiene program director affects attitudes toward the program, the acceptance of the personnel and dental hygiene students, and the support the program receives. The rapid growth of professional education in colleges is cause for grave concern in many institutions of higher education. Faculty and administrators ask, "Is dental hygiene just another vocational program seeking status? What does the dental hygiene program have to offer the college? Should a dental hygiene program be offered in a four-year institution and award a baccalaureate degree? Should the baccalaureate degree be entry level into the profession? Should dental hygiene change from two-year associate degree programs to four-year baccalaureate degree programs? Will dental hygiene lower the scholastic standards of the college? What does dental hygiene expect from other departments?" These are all legitimate concerns and questions that are constantly raised and which the director must evaluate and answer.

The role of the director varies depending on the organization in which the dental hygiene program is located. As universities and colleges move toward greater centralization of authority and decision making, the director's authority may lie at the level of middle or lower management. Most directors in charge of individual faculties and programs are considered middle management, although some are considered lower level. The amount of authority or autonomy determines the level of leadership. The director as an academic administrator is responsible for the following functions: administration of curriculum, administration of faculty, student personnel services, administration of the budget, research, collaboration, and evaluation of the program.

Because the program director's job responsibilities vary from physical plant operations to future planning for the program, and everything in between, no leadership class or degree can replace experience. A dental hygienist planning to become a program director should take management courses such as the one-day seminars offered on leadership or supervisory skills or courses within a university MBA program. Stay up to date in your reading, including nursing management literature and the suggested reading listed at the end of this chapter and others. I was given a copy of *Educational Administration in Nursing* (Gallagher, 1965) when I was first appointed as a director and I continue to use this book as a reference. In addition, attending professional meetings, such as the annual session of the American Association of Dental Schools and National Dental Directors' meeting, helps me to learn and stay up to date.

The dental hygiene director must handle many responsibilities simultaneously—that of chief executive officer of the program, leader in the profession, chief financial officer of the program, mentor to less-experienced faculty and peers, writer, researcher, and change agent. It is the balance of these various roles, as well as the skill that the director uses in fulfilling them, that makes the difference between a director who is successful and one who is mediocre.

# ADMINISTRATION OF CURRICULUM

The greatest responsibility of the program director is the development of the curriculum. Although curriculum development is a continuing responsibility of the faculty, the director's understanding of educational concepts and attitude toward newer concepts in dental hygiene education greatly influence the attitude of faculty. The director needs a broad view of professional education and should be alert to educational trends. Because the director has an overall responsibility for curriculum and development, and has an opportunity to study the complete scope of curricula in the college, the director generally has broader views concerning professional curricula. It is the responsibility of the director to guide the faculty toward implementing new concepts in the curriculum.

## Philosophy and Objectives of the Curriculum

The philosophy of the college reflects the beliefs of those who comprise the college. The philosophy and objectives of the dental hygiene program should be developed by the faculty of the program, should be in harmony with, or at least closely related to, the philosophy of the institution of which it is a part, and should mirror the philosophy of the dental hygiene program. It is the faculty's responsibility to write objectives that identify the knowledge, attitudes, and skills students need to become professional dental hygienists.

## Organization of Curriculum

Once the objectives of the program have been developed and approved by the faculty and the administration of the college, the next step is to organize the curriculum. Faculty members should not be the sole participants in curriculum development. There should be students on the curriculum committee. They can make a significant contribution to the development of their educational program. In addition, the public also has a place in curriculum development. The "public" may include practicing dental hygienists, trustees, other people within the college, representatives from other dental facilities, or community agencies at large. As in any educational program, the curriculum committee of the dental hygiene program plays a distinctive role. The structure of the dental hygiene curriculum committee may vary with the size of the program and faculty. In smaller programs the committee usually consists of about eight people—faculty representation from the basic sciences, dental sciences, dental hygiene sciences, students, and one or two community leaders. The chair of the curriculum committee, usually a person other than the director, should be well informed about educational trends and curriculum research and have leadership ability.

The program director is responsible for gaining financial support for the program and for gaining support from central administration, college personnel, and the community for the curriculum. The director is involved in deciding what resources will be made available to implement the curriculum plan and who will teach specific courses and in the refereeing of curriculum controversy. Sometimes power struggles among the faculty center on curricular issues, so the director must be clearly involved in the curricular building process.

Curriculum development and revision is a continuous cycle. It is something that should be included in every long-range plan and should take place every five to seven years. In this way, the program will not become stagnant and will always be looking toward the future and the necessary changes that need to be made so that the graduates are prepared for the future.

## Selection of Learning Experiences

Objectives should be defined in terms of behaviors that students are expected to demonstrate. Learning experiences, or activities carried out by students, should be based upon those objectives. Students attain the objectives of the dental hygiene program through the learning experiences selected by the faculty. In selecting learning experiences, the faculty must think in terms of those experiences that will give students an opportunity to practice the behaviors stated in the objectives, and in terms of content that will give them the basic knowledge, understanding, and appreciation to prepare them to become professional dental hygienists.

The teaching methodology used in the classroom is critical. It is important that the faculty keep abreast of new teaching methodologies as they are researched and proven successful. Problem-based learning is an important new educational trend. Students should be exposed to client situations and problems they can solve themselves to internalize the information. Using new teaching methods can also help keep the classroom interesting. In designing classroom teaching, use state-of-the-art instructional media such as interactive videotapes and computer-simulated instruction. Whenever possible, use new methods and find the resources to support the development of new instructional materials.

## Administrative Coordination of Curriculum

Coordination of the ongoing operations of the dental hygiene program embraces all aspects of the administrative process. It is important to make sure that the dental hygiene program offers a rich mix of learning experiences in the humanities and social sciences, as well as natural science. Courses in the program should be planned on an academic term basis. Assignment of credit for courses and for clinical practice should be in accordance with the policies of the institution. The director needs to make sure that the curriculum includes carefully selected learning experiences that develop students' competency in essential areas of dental hygiene. Specialization should be reserved for graduate study.

## Continuous Evaluation

Evaluation is an integral part of curriculum development, providing for continued improvement of the dental hygiene program. Evaluation can guide faculty in the selection of learning experiences. Students should participate in curriculum evaluation because the curriculum affects them directly. Evaluation forms can be developed internally or adapted from other dental hygiene programs willing to share theirs and should address course content, faculty teaching, and current learning experiences. Faculty should conduct follow-up studies of alumni opinions and progress to determine to what extent the objectives of the program have been realized. This type of evaluation is called outcome assessment and is required by most accrediting agencies and organizations of higher education. Evaluation of the dental hygiene program also serves the purpose of making everyone aware of the fact that the curriculum is current and that the program is responding to changing needs. Evaluation provides for continued improvement of the curriculum. As students and faculty participate in evaluating learning outcomes, the information gathered can be utilized to further improve the curriculum and program.

# ADMINISTRATION OF FACULTY

The quality of the faculty determines the quality of the dental hygiene program. One of the most vital functions of the director is therefore to appoint able, well-prepared faculty members, for which the recruitment process is a major task. It is essential that the director not only select faculty carefully, but retain good faculty and provide for their professional development.

The director faces a number of challenges in selecting qualified faculty members for teaching. The schools with more money, more facilities and resources, more opportunities for success, and more prestige tend to attract faculty members more readily than do schools with limited resources. Another challenge in recruiting quality faculty members is the "big university" image that perpetuates itself, particularly among faculty members who received degrees from major universities. The big university concept encompasses a light teaching load, with an emphasis on research, teaching advanced subject matter, and building a reputation through publishing. All directors should take into consideration some of these factors in recruiting and talking to new faculty members.

In addition to selection and appointment of well-prepared faculty, there should be adequate numbers of faculty in order that the program can operate effectively. When talking to individuals interested in a faculty position, I ask them to consider whether teaching is their primary focus or whether their interests include teaching, research, and service. I also ask them to consider the different demands of a university versus a community college. In this way, a potential faculty member's interest can be compared to the institution's objectives.

## Faculty Selection and Recruitment

In selecting faculty, it is important that the description of the duties and qualifications required for each job be well defined by the administration. It is also important to have a long-range plan for recruitment of faculty. When developing this plan, the director should consider the required numbers and qualifications of faculty members needed due to retirement, resignation, or expansion of the program. When writing job descriptions, it is important to consider the types of courses that each faculty member will be teaching, the committees on which they will serve, the type of service activities in which they will be involved, and most important, the expertise required to fulfill their responsibilities. Having a plan and job description will serve to facilitate the development of the announcement of each faculty position opening and the conduction of the interview. Recruiting and selecting faculty takes a considerable amount of time due to mandatory institutional guidelines set up by the administration and delineated in the policies of the school. Usually a selection committee is appointed consisting of administration and faculty members. The remainder of the recruitment process consists of advertising the position in a number of national, state, and local journals or newspapers, setting a deadline for application submission, and scheduling the actual interviews.

Some ideas for recruiting new faculty include establishing working relationships with graduate programs in your area and staying in touch with alumni of your program who have expressed an interest in becoming faculty members. It is a good idea to work with other colleges so that when you send out the advertisement of positions you can also send announcements to them. It is typical to receive 20 to 30 applications for a given position. Send a letter to all applicants, acknowledging receipt of their application. The search committee or director then evaluates the qualifications of each applicant, using an appraisal form. In addition to the application, recommendation letters from former employers, transcripts from graduate schools, curriculum vitae, plus any other information, should be evaluated. The next step is to select the top three or five applicants and arrange for these candidates to visit the campus for personal interviews. The interview provides the faculty, the director, and the administration the opportunity to discover the candidates' attitudes, philosophy, previous teaching experiences, ability to express themselves, and ability to gain insight into their understanding of dental hygiene educational concepts. During the one- to two-day visit, it is important that the candidate meet not only with the director, but also with faculty members, students, and administrators of the college. After all the candidates are interviewed, a final decision can be made.

Usually all college or university handbooks or policy manuals contain specifications of requirements for appointment to the college. Many detail the procedures to follow, the requirements of the faculty, the appointing authority, length of appointment, guidelines toward tenure, and the background necessary for appointment. The recommendation of a specific candidate is then made to the president, who in turn forwards the documentation to the board of regents or board of trustees. Upon authorization of the appointment, the director sends the candidate a letter of appointment. The transition is closed upon receipt of the candidate's written acceptance of the appointment.

## Faculty Development

The director must always take steps to promote the continuous professional growth and development of faculty members. Meaningful professional development increases the effectiveness of faculty and, additionally, is a successful method of retaining them. Quality of education is obviously influenced by the quality of faculty. Appointees to large universities are usually required to have a doctorate degree.

Because dental hygiene has a scarcity of doctorates, the majority of the dental hygiene faculty will have master's degrees and so differ in their educational preparation from other faculty in the college or university. Preparation at the master's level does not adequately prepare individuals for the multitude of responsibilities in institutions of higher education. A well-defined program will therefore assist faculty in the attainment of a doctorate degree and allow time for this achievement.

An orientation program should be provided for new faculty members. It should be very carefully planned in order to accomplish its purpose of presenting information about the university, its personnel benefits, and the dental hygiene program. The orientation program should be more detailed for the inexperienced faculty member than for the experienced teacher, who only needs assistance bridging the gap between former employment and the new position. The orientation program, of course, will vary from program to program. Some are set up by the actual dental hygiene program, and some include input from the faculty development office of the university or community college.

The faculty development process may be continuous and called *in-service*. The in-service program may consist of experiences with course development, instruction on writing syllabi, establishing remedial programs, or educational technology courses on problem-based learning. A number of colleges and universities have formal programs in faculty development for various faculty members and are not limited to dental hygiene.

The program at the University of Colorado Health Sciences Center is a good example. The educational resource department offers two to three courses per month in educational methodology, including techniques in developing audiovisuals, writing better test questions, using problem-based learning, and developing a teaching portfolio. A number of programs have also established a mentoring program wherein a new faculty member is assigned to an established faculty member to develop skills in research, classroom preparation and presentation, and committee work. A mentoring program is an excellent idea in larger schools or programs with more than six faculty members. The program can be very effective for faculty members who are just starting teaching or for a faculty member who has been teaching in another university.

At the University of Colorado, we use faculty contracts. During the summer prior to the start of the new academic year, each faculty member prepares a contract that includes course goals, necessary changes, and required resources (additional slides, videotapes, or other visual aids). The contract also details research activities—funding needs, articles to be published from previous research, and new research projects. The contract also covers service to the associations or organizations in which faculty are members and continuing education courses they plan to present in the coming year. In addition, they identify areas of national interest, such as committee activities in the dental hygiene education section of the American Association of Dental Schools or the American Dental Hygienists' Association.

I review the completed contracts at the beginning of the school year before meeting with each faculty member to review, discuss, and sign the contract. This contract is then used at the year-end compensation review (for salary increase, promotion, or merit review by the administration of the school). A positive evaluation at the end of the year is given to those faculty members who have published a number of articles, given presentations at national meetings, presented continuing education courses, or had a strong service component. Year-end evaluations also acknowledge outstanding peer reviews from classroom observations, plus outstanding evaluations from students regarding the faculty member's presentations and course development. The contract is used to evaluate whether the faculty member has accomplished the stated goals and the member's individual growth over a period of time.

## Promotion of Faculty

Terms of appointment should be clearly stated. The faculty member may be appointed for the current year, for two or three years, or for permanent tenure. Usually younger and new faculty members are appointed for a limited term to give the educational institution the opportunity to observe whether the faculty member can adapt to the philosophy of the dental hygiene program. Appointment is usually made at the level of "instructor" for younger faculty members and "assistant professor" for those with several years of experience and some publications. The first three years may be considered a probationary period in many institutions for those appointed at the rank of instructor. Some of the larger universities may even count the first three years of a faculty member's appointment at the assistant professor level as a probationary period.

Community colleges sometimes do not have individual ranks. Everyone is appointed at the entry level, and their titles do not change as they are given longer terms of appointment. Probationary periods vary for tenure, but most colleges have adopted the recommendations of the American Association of University Professors and the American Association of American Colleges and have chosen a seven-year probationary period to obtain tenure. During this period, the faculty member may be promoted from the rank of instructor to assistant professor and must have developed the credentials required by the institution for tenure. At my university, research, teaching, and service activities are considered.

Research must be meritorious, and teaching and service performance must be outstanding for a member to be awarded tenure. Meritorious research means that a requisite amount of research has been completed and published in refereed journals. Outstanding in teaching indicates that the faculty member is considered an expert in his field and that he has received excellent evaluations from students. The faculty member's teaching portfolio must include examples of teaching syllabi, videotapes, and/or textbooks written. Service consists of being involved in national, state, and local association activities; having a statewide or national reputation; presenting continuing education courses; presenting at national meetings; and being an active participant in schoolwide and university committees.

The director of the program, in addition to working with the faculty and giving them time to do their research so they can be tenured and promoted, also needs to deal with faculty compensation. This can be by an increase in salary, granting of sabbatical leave, or promotion from instructor to assistant professor. The director should inform the faculty members regarding the salary scale for each rank and how each rank is rewarded or evaluated for a raise in salary. Some universities do not have salary scales; the money allocated for raises is given to the program and the administrator can award it according to merit. Merit increases usually range from 1% to 5%, depending upon faculty performance during the past year.

In our program, salary increases relate to the contracts that faculty members developed at the beginning of the academic year. Also in my program, and within the School of Dentistry, the faculty are rated for publications and research they have done in the past year, how many national offices or committees they have served on, student and peer evaluations of their teaching, how well they are doing in developing their teaching portfolio, and their service activities. Faculty members are graded in these areas and are ranked as meeting expectations, exceeding expectations, or outstanding. All promotions to assistant professor, associate professor, full professor, and tenure are done through school committees and the administration. Committees are assigned the task of evaluating the faculty in accordance with the university and/or community college policies.

# STUDENT SERVICES

Student support services aid individual students in developing their abilities or potential. The major responsibilities for administrating and coordinating student support services falls under the dean of student services, who might be referred to as an associate or assistant dean of academic and student affairs. The dental hygiene director, however, is responsible for functions such as participating in the overall recruitment and admission of students, for disseminating information, for working with other administrative personnel in promoting student welfare, for maintaining a system of records, and for counseling students so they may use the services more effectively. The director must interpret policies and practices to the faculty members and secure their support for policies that have been adopted by the college.

Student personnel services have expanded in number and scope to keep pace with the growing number of students and the variety of problems that occur. The ranges and type of services vary with the size and educational philosophy of the college or university. These services may range from preadmission testing and counseling to placement services for the alumni, with a wide variety of services available to students during their enrollment in college. The dental hygiene program is governed by the policies of the educational institution in matters such as selection, admission, academic progression, and orientation. Students in the program are college students first and dental hygiene students second. They have problems similar to students majoring in other disciplines and therefore have similar needs for student support services. While student support services are mainly conducted and coordinated by individuals within the college or university, the director has a wide range of responsibilities in promoting student welfare.

## Recruitment and Selection of Students

The director is responsible for the recruitment, selection, and preparation of professional dental hygienists. When college representatives are invited to high school career days, the dental hygiene director is usually asked to attend to impart information about the program to prospective dental hygiene students. In addition, visits to college campuses around the area will also help identify and recruit prospective students into the program. Other faculty members should also be asked to participate in recruitment activities. Whoever attends the college or the high school career days needs to be acquainted with the programs, goals, requirements for admission into the programs, costs, scholarships and loans, residence facilities, and future and present opportunities for dental hygienists. The director will work with the admissions office of the college or university to make sure that mailings go out, including recruitment brochures to teachers, predental advisers in the high schools, and colleges and counselors around the area.

The admissions committee is probably one of the most important committees because it selects the students for the program. Admissions selection is based upon grades, either in high school or college, entrance test results, interviews, and references from instructors. The admissions committee should include faculty members from different disciplines, alumni, and students, so that many viewpoints are represented to form an objective analysis of the applicants. The methods of selection vary in different colleges and community colleges. Some admit all graduates of accredited state secondary schools regardless of the scholastic achievement or program of studies pursued. Test results are used for selection for scholarship and to guide the students after admission. In some programs, the science grade point average in college or the overall grade point average are used as criteria in selection. The mix of in-state to out-of-state applicants and the numbers of people that need to be selected to meet the college's commitment to the affirmative action plan must always be taken into consideration.

## Student Orientation

In addition to recruitment and admissions into the program, the director cooperates with student support services in planning an orientation program for new students. Our orientation program consists of registration, school photos, a campus tour, library orientation, locker assignment, completion of the registration paperwork, meeting with the financial aid officers, meeting with the faculty, and the issuing of instruments to the students. In addition to discussing the policies of the school, we discuss the Student American Dental Hygienists' Association (SADHA) program, the student council, and class offices. Student health services are discussed and student physicals are conducted during orientation.

Improving student welfare, financial aid, and scholarships for students in the dental hygiene program should be a high priority for the director. Soliciting funds and establishing criteria for scholarships for the dental hygiene students are also responsibilities of the director. The director works with the financial aid office so that students who are in need of work-study, grants, or loans will be able to get the proper paperwork completed. The director also needs to become familiar with other sources of scholarships for students, such as the scholarships supported by the American Dental Hygienists' Association Institute for Oral Health and the American Dental Association scholarships for dental hygiene students.

Students occasionally need academic counseling, which is the responsibility of faculty members. Each faculty member serves as an adviser to a selected number of students concerning such matters as sequence of courses, scholastic progress, study habits, and graduation requirements. When necessary, the adviser refers students to the administration for further counseling, referral, or assignment of tutors.

## STUDENT RECORDS

The director is responsible for maintaining a system of records for the program. To work with students, faculty must keep records for each student enrolled in the program. These records should consist of the admissions information, their high school or college transcripts, preadmission testing, interviews, educational background, and experiences. Records maintained for each student include scholastic achievement records, academic standing, behavioral or academic advising, honors earned, offices held, national board scores, and regional clinical examination results. We have a release form that is also kept in the student's file. Students sign this form to give the faculty permission to give references for future employment and/or graduate school. All faculty members need to understand the importance and confidentiality of the data in the students' files. The director interprets policy regarding record keeping and makes sure that faculty and staff support the policies of the college.

## ADMINISTRATION OF THE BUDGET

The budget defines the limits of financial support for the educational institution and as such impacts the scope and quality of the institution's program. It affects policy that determines the quality and size of faculty, potential number of students, and thus the quality of instruction. It determines the amount and type of equipment, library and laboratory resources, physical facilities, and other resources that will be available for instruction and research.

The budget, following the institution's strategic plan, gives direction for action. The annual budget is also affected by institutionwide projects. With increased college enrollments, increased interest in research, and a need for expansion of college facilities, it is becoming increasingly important to make long-term budget projections. Educational institutions are beginning to make five- year or ten-year budget projections.

One of the major problems institutions of higher education face is financing. Because few colleges can finance themselves on the basis of money collected from tuition fees alone, other sources of funds must be sought to balance the expenditures, both educational and noneducational. Private institutions derive added income from endowments and gifts; public institutions from state appropriations, gifts, and grants. Inflation, expanding educational services, increasing enrollments, uncertainty of sources of funds, and expanding requirements to accommodate increasing enrollment are some of the financial problems faced by institutions of higher education. Educational institutions are often short of money, resulting in problems allocating monies among the various departments or divisions of the college and other competing requests.

## Management of a Dental Hygiene Program Budget

The director plays a key role in the management of the program's budget. Community colleges, colleges, and universities all have different budgeting mechanisms. Directors of dental hygiene programs can be responsible for their own budget preparation, or this may be the responsibility of the director of the allied health program. The administration of the budget will be different in each situation. One important factor is that the administrator not only has the responsibility but the authority to plan the budget, to make budget recommendations needed to manage the program well, and to approve resources allocation.

The budget should be in accordance with the philosophy of the institution and the support that the educational program receives. A well-organized faculty plans its instructional program for the coming year and makes their recommendations for the fiscal year, requesting supplies, equipment, facilities, and library and research resources. Sufficient funds should be requested to support a sound educational program, to provide for faculty development, to provide for the expansion of course offerings, to attract and hold qualified faculty members, and to provide for proper physical facilities, supplies, and resources for instruction. If the dental hygiene program is a division within a department of a college, the director turns in the budget requests, recommendations, and justification to the dean of the larger unit. The dean integrates the various departmental budget requests into the larger unit for submission to the university at large.

## Record Keeping

After the budget has been approved, management of the budget becomes the director's responsibility. Using computers simplifies this task. The director's budgetary control includes approving expenditure requests and keeping detailed records of all requests or actions. The budget must be flexible, with provisions for contingencies. The director's budgetary control allows rapid and convenient checking against the ledgers of the institution's finance office. The finance officer sends periodic statements to each program that show the budget appropriations, expenditures, encumbrances in detail, and the available balance for future expenditures. The director's detailed records allow rapid analysis and comparison of the finance department's report.

## Financial Reporting System

Budgets are broken down into categories depending on the institution. These may include salaries, the operating fund, equipment, clinic support, travel, and equipment repair. Salaries for faculty and support staff may include benefits, insurance, FICA payment, disability, medical and dental insurance, and retirement. The operating fund includes the telephone, office supplies, educational support materials, development courses for faculty or staff, and registration for attending meetings.

Equipment is usually a separate category because it is a high dollar expenditure and the finance officer has to approve the purchases. Items included in the equipment budget might include computer equipment, ultrasonic instruments, or dental chairs. Equipment repair might be a separate category and would pertain to service contracts with vendors to repair dental equipment, computers, or copy machines.

The clinic support budget covers all supplies for teaching clinical and pre-clinical programs, for example, instruments, charting forms, toothbrushes, and the like. Some colleges have a separate budget for travel, which allows faculty to attend professional and research meetings and other travel for faculty development. The director's immediate supervisor usually retains the responsibility of accounting for these expenditures.

## Income Estimates

Clinic fees are an excellent source of income. In some dental hygiene programs, the fees collected for client care services are allocated to the dental hygiene program budget. In other programs, the state requires the program to generate a certain amount of income from the clinical program, but the income is not credited directly to the dental hygiene program and they are not able to use those additional resources. Clinic fees should be realistic. Some programs are still charging $5 or $10 a clinic visit, whereas other programs are charging half of what is charged in the community. For example, the charge for an adult prophylaxis in a dental hygiene program may be $25 compared to $50 in the community. Scaling and root planing for quadrants might be $200 in the dental hygiene school, compared to $600 in the private sector. Whatever the resources, remember to be futuristic. Your students need to know how to manage dental hygiene services, not only treatment, but also fees.

Other sources of funding are small grants to the college that might allow for a one-time purchase of new equipment. Also, development funds may be available to faculty members to cover the cost of travel and lodging to enable them to attend or give presentations at national meetings. The profits from continuing education courses presented by the program should be deposited into a development account and be available for faculty to use to conduct research or attend seminars. Consider contacting local and state foundations to request grant money to conduct research or to design new programs. There are also grants available from the National Institutes of Health. Smaller grants from the American Dental Hygienists' Association Institute for Oral Health, Oral-B Laboratories, the Procter & Gamble Company, and other companies are excellent sources of funding.

## RESEARCH

Research is advancement of knowledge and is part of the mission of institutions of higher education. Dental hygiene faculty members in universities or colleges are involved in research along with faculty members from other departments. Dental hygiene programs in community colleges place more emphasis on service and education. The research responsibilities of the director may not apply to all programs.

Like other professionals, dental hygienists have shown increased interest in research. To attain and maintain its professional status, dental hygiene must recognize and develop, through research, a specialized body of dental hygiene knowledge. Only recently have dental hygiene investigations dealt with the practice of dental hygiene. Early studies were mainly surveys concerned with the dental hygienist's attitudes and education and dental hygiene organization and administration. Dental hygiene took much of its clinical research from the periodontal or dental research until recently, because dental hygienists had not been prepared to do scientific investigations. Programs had to be developed to prepare them to do research. Faculty members in graduate and doctorate programs have led us forward, and more individuals are now prepared to conduct research.

The director plays an important role in stimulating interest in research, in advocating and promoting measures that will support investigation in dental hygiene service, and in dental hygiene education. The director must be aware of sources of funding for research, must understand research findings, and must make adequate use of these findings to improve the dental hygiene education program. The director is responsible for creating a climate conducive to seeking knowledge, where faculty members explore and use research findings. The director should promote faculty participation in research, initiate research projects, and participate in them. The faculty should be encouraged to participate and to publish their research findings.

The faculty at the University at Colorado have been very successful in receiving research grants. They also have a valuable network that enables them to conduct research with faculty from other departments. They have been successful in presenting their findings at the International Association for Dental Research annual meetings and other research forums and publishing the results in refereed journals. As mentioned in the discussion on faculty promotion, the participation and success of the faculty in the area of research is one of the criteria for promotion and tenure within a university. The director of the university-based program needs to make research a high priority in the program so that faculty will have the necessary resources, allotted time, and facilities to conduct their research.

## NETWORKING, COLLABORATION, AND INTERRELATIONS

The dental hygiene program is involved in a variety of relationships with other instructional units within the educational institution, with dental service agencies and health agencies, with other institutions of higher learning, and within the profession. Cooperation among the instructional units within the university will determine the extent of collaboration with your instructional program. It is important to establish good communication with all instructional units. Formal linkages should be established with the health service agencies and dental facilities to enable student rotations and other sorts of collaborative activities. Working with other schools of dental hygiene around the country is necessary to ensure that dental hygiene programs utilize the resources of higher education to the fullest extent possible. Collaboration between the dental hygiene profession and other health professions is needed if the dental hygiene profession is to advance.

## Collaboration Within the Educational Institution

The policies of the college determine the extent of cooperation among instructional units. Each unit is responsible for its own operation, although dental hygiene courses can be taught by other units. An example is basic science. Without close collaboration, a situation might develop where one of the liberal arts units or basic sciences units decided to make major changes in its courses without consulting the dental hygiene program. This could be problematic, especially if it involved a scheduling change. It is essential that there be coordination among the instructional units.

Much of the necessary coordination can be accomplished through committee structure, by involving people from the other units on the dental hygiene curriculum committee. If they meet on a regular basis, and a unit is considering changes, the pending changes could be discussed at a meeting, permitting coordination between units.

Collaboration is extremely important for the start-up dental hygiene program. In designing the basic science courses for the science unit, such as chemistry, biology, and head and neck anatomy, it is important to work with that unit to design courses for dental hygiene students only. This is essential so that the dental hygiene students are not placed in a general chemistry course that would not give them the necessary biochemistry background required for additional courses in the dental hygiene curriculum.

It is important that the program director be a member of central councils and committees of the university in order to have an opportunity to be part of the policy making of the college. The director should take every opportunity afforded to participate on these committees and to have the dental hygiene faculty represented on universitywide and health sciences centerwide committees. Participation on college committees gives the administrator or faculty member opportunities to network and to be involved in matters such as budget allocation, public relations, tenure issues, scholastic standards, legislative issues, and outcome assessments for the entire university or center.

It is also important that the program director and the faculty be involved in the faculty organization of the university. Volunteering to serve on relevant committees and participating in faculty meetings are positive factors, not only within the program's school, but also within the health sciences center or the entire university. Any time that the director or faculty members can let people know about the dental hygiene program—whether with the library, learning resources, educational support, or program directors of other allied health groups—both its support and knowledge base increase.

## Collaboration with the Community

Programs in dental hygiene exist for the purpose of preparing dental hygienists who are capable of giving the quality and quantity of dental hygiene care demanded by the community. Opportunities for collaboration exist with dental health programs or through the community area hospitals that have dental facilities. Examples would be the Veterans' Administration Hospital, city hospitals, children's hospitals, dental clinics within neighborhood health units, nursing homes that offer oral health services, health centers for the homeless that have dental facilities, and school education programs that have oral health components.

Collaborate with any groups or agencies that offer dental care or education programs. Your only involvement may be to offer guidance, or you may establish extramural rotations for students to work in some of these facilities as part of student enrichment programs. It is good public relations to be involved with programs that receive community, state, or federal support and promote health throughout your state.

In our dental hygiene program, second-year students can choose to spend a half a day a week in many different practice settings. They can choose to participate in oral health education programs in the classroom, a sealant program at one of our junior high schools, a clinical program with the handicapped or developmentally disabled population (through the National Foundation of Dentistry for the Handicapped), deliver dental hygiene care in one of the many hospital programs, or work with the homeless or the geriatric population to refine their skills.

## Collaboration with Professionals

Evidence of collaboration within the dental hygiene profession is found at all levels—internationally, nationally, regionally, and locally. The need for collaboration within the profession cannot be overemphasized. For the dental hygiene profession to advance and realize its full potential, dental hygienists must collaborate with the other health professions (nursing, dentistry, and medicine).

Through international collaboration, we are able to better understand the oral health needs and delivery systems of other countries. The number of foreign dental hygienists coming to the United States has increased. Dental hygiene programs can be resources for foreign graduates to assist them in obtaining the necessary credentials required to apply for licensing in the United States. Directors of U.S. dental hygiene programs have been asked to assist in starting dental hygiene programs in other countries.

Dental hygiene activity at the national level is primarily through the American Dental Hygienists' Association (ADHA) and the American Association of Dental Schools (AADS). It is important for the director and other faculty members to be active, participating members of these associations and receive their journals and newsletters. Attending national meetings is important for all dental hygiene administrators and educators. They should also be active members in research associations, such as the American Association of Dental Research or the International Association for Dental Research. All of these organizations offer opportunities for continuing education, professional development, grants and research funding, and the exchange of research findings.

State dental hygiene associations are active in offering workshops and programs for practicing, licensed dental hygienists, in addition to working in the legislative arena to continue to advance the profession of dental hygiene. Faculty involvement at the state level can be quite valuable, although some institutions have policies restricting legislative activity of faculty members. The faculty at the University of Colorado Dental Hygiene Program has been very supportive of the legislative initiatives of the Colorado Dental Hygienists Association. Faculty activity at local and state professional meetings may involve serving as members of the House of Delegates, presenting continuing education courses, assisting with course design and/or development, and attending meetings as a member. It is very important to be seen at these meetings and to be there to support the professional association.

Offering continuing education courses, through the adult education department or other appropriate departments, for dental hygienists should be part of the mission of all the dental hygiene programs so that the programs support life-long learning. A college with clinical facilities can offer both clinical and didactic courses because it has resources that local professional organizations lack. The dental hygiene program can also be instrumental in attracting national leaders in dental hygiene to provide courses on the latest research. The planning, organization, and marketing for continuing education courses take a great deal of time, but the rewards are evident as you fulfill the mission of your college and help advance your profession.

## Educational Initiatives

An educational leader plays an important role in shaping policies for dental hygiene education that have implications, not only for one dental hygiene program, but for the region and for the nation. In different parts of the country, groups meet regionally and plan for that area in order to be more effective. It is important that regional plans be addressed by the college and the dental hygiene program. In Ohio and some western states (e.g., California, Oregon, Washington), strong regional groups of directors and faculty meet to participate in long-range planning regarding needs of programs, sharing new technology in education, telecommunications, and future direction.

Due to the rapidly expanding knowledge and technology, and changing social and educational needs of society, it is important to work with the other programs within the state. The increasing need for a diversified system of higher education, the scarcity of prepared faculty, and the increasing cost of higher education have made us aware of the fact that coordination and long-range planning can solve some of the problems that confront our colleges and our profession. The trend is toward long-range planning and coordination of activities among institutions. In the past, there was probably some competition between programs, but today cooperation has become more the norm. Cooperation can involve sharing course outlines, faculty, or educational methodology.

The University of Colorado shares library resources (e.g., videotapes) with the other associate degree programs nearby for a nominal fee and cost of postage. Since we are in a dental school, we also share research information from our university. In our state, the faculty and directors meet once a year in coordination with our state dental hygiene meeting. Each school rotates in sharing the responsibility of planning the meeting and the agenda items. We have found this to be an effective way to share resources and to do some long-range planning for the future of the dental hygiene programs within our state. We have also included schools from neighboring states because they do not have some of the resources that we do.

It is important for the director to become familiar with state coordinating agencies that seek to improve the quality of instruction by decreasing costs that originally resulted from duplication of major functions of institutions and by centralizing programs in institutions that have adequate facilities and resources. For example, in Colorado there were duplications in two or three of our state universities and the Commission on Higher Education made recommendations to eliminate some of those programs to reduce costs.

Long-range planning for higher education in a state must take into consideration dentistry, nursing, medicine, pharmacy, and other health professions. It is important that the dental hygiene program and/or state professional association has representation on statewide planning groups that look at educational issues and also health service agency issues. In the future, these agencies may be looking at funding issues and healthcare reform.

In addition, it is important to work with the board of dental or dental hygiene examiners, as they are the licensing agency for the graduates of your program. In Colorado, there are dentists, dental hygienists, and consumers on the board. The role of the director of a dental hygiene program is to network with members of the board, since rules and regulations governing the practice of dental hygiene do change. It is a good practice to know your members and to work with them when they need information on dental hygiene practice. Board meetings are open to the public. Attend meetings to give testimony and to support to your profession.

## EVALUATION OF THE PROGRAM

Evaluation of the dental hygiene program is a continuous process. Many instruments and devices are used to evaluate various aspects of the education offered. For example, teacher-made tests and standardized tests measure student achievement, reflecting on the quality of the instruction and the quality of the curriculum. Other members of the health professions, students, dentists, physicians, the public, and faculty may participate in the evaluative process. While the opinion of these groups may not be regarded as scientific evaluation, it is nevertheless an expression of their estimate of the quality of the program. The college participates in the appraisal of its educational offerings. For example, the university collects data on students' grades in each instructional unit, data concerning students on academic probation, and data concerning those who have attained scholastic distinction. These are some of the instruments used in evaluating the quality of the dental hygiene program.

The results of national board examinations and specific regional clinical examination are used as an evaluation of the program in outcomes assessment. In addition, graduates are asked to evaluate their curriculum in relationship to their positions after they have graduated. Additional measures of outcomes include alumni surveys three years after graduation to evaluate how well the program prepared them to practice dental hygiene. The employers of those same graduates are also asked to evaluate the curriculum in terms of how it prepared the graduates for the practice. Outcome assessments are being done for different accreditation agencies and for some of the commissions on higher education.

The agency that accredits dental hygiene programs is the Commission on Dental Accreditation (CODA) of the American Dental Association. CODA is the accrediting body for dental schools, dental hygiene, dental assisting and laboratory technology programs, plus specialty graduate programs in dentistry. The commission is responsible for the site visit and approval of programs on a seven-year rotation.

As part of the accrediting process, the program must complete and submit a self-evaluation report to the commission prior to the seven-year site visit. Guidelines for dental hygiene programs are approved and must be followed in submitting the self-evaluation report. Site visit teams spend approximately two days on campus visiting the dental hygiene program. The team of evaluators consists of representatives from other dental hygiene programs, staff representatives from the commission, and usually a member of the local state board of dental or dental hygiene examiners. The site visit and the actual completion of the self-evaluation should be looked upon as a positive experience. The director of the program should give the faculty full support and encouragement to determine objectively the strengths and weaknesses of the program and to make recommendations for improvement in the program prior to the actual site visit.

In addition, the entire university is evaluated by one of the six regional accrediting agencies in the United States: New England Association of Colleges and Secondary Schools, Middle States Association of Colleges and Secondary Schools, North Central Association of Colleges and Secondary Schools, Southern Association of Colleges and Secondary Schools, Northwest Association of Secondary and Higher Schools, and Western College Association. Membership in these agencies is voluntary. Each agency establishes criteria for the evaluation of institutions in its region. It reviews those institutions periodically and publishes a list of institutions that it has accredited. Representatives from each of the six regional accreditation agencies make up the National Committee of Regional Accreditation Agencies of the United States. Regional accrediting agencies are concerned with appraising the total activities of institutions of higher learning and the safeguarding of quality of liberal education, the foundation of professional groups and colleges and universities.

## *Review Questions*

1. List the seven functions for which the director of an academic program is responsible.

2. Write a job description for the director of a dental hygiene program.

3. Assume you want to teach in a dental hygiene program and eventually to become a program director. What personal goals would be required to accomplish your objective?

4. Define what a dental hygiene program's commitment should be to teaching, research, and service.

5. What mechanisms are available for recruiting new faculty members for a dental hygiene program?

6. What components of student services does the director of a dental hygiene program manage?

7. What expense categories might be included in the yearly budget of a dental hygiene program?

8. Describe the evaluation processes that a dental hygiene program must go through.

9. Give at least five examples of ways to accomplish outcomes assessment for a dental hygiene program.

10. In your area, what community agencies or facilities offering oral health services might be interested in collaboration with your dental hygiene program?

11. Which of the professional associations mentioned in this chapter are you a member of? Which would you join in the future and for what reasons?

12. What research questions would you investigate that would advance the dental hygiene body of knowledge?

## SUGGESTED READING

American Dental Association, Commission on Dental Accreditation. (1992). *Accreditation standards for dental hygiene education programs.* Chicago: ADA.

Bennis, W. (1989). *On becoming a leader.* Reading, MA: Addison-Wesley.

Covey, S. R. (1989). *The seven habits of highly effective people.* New York: Simon and Schuster.

Creswell, J. W., et al. (1990). *The academic chairperson's handbook.* Lincoln: University of Nebraska Press.

DePree, M. (1989). *Leadership is an art.* New York: Doubleday.

LeBoeuf, M. (1985). *The greatest management principles in the world.* New York: Berkeley Books.

Roberts, W. (1987). *Leadership secrets of Attila the Hun.* New York: Warner Books.

Rombert, E., ed. (1990). *Outcomes assessment handbook.* Washington, D.C.: American Association of Dental Schools.

## REFERENCES

Gallagher, A. H. (1965). *Educational administration in nursing.* New York: Macmillan Co.

*Candy B. Ross*

# CHAPTER 12

# Oral Healthcare Products Industry

## *Objectives*

After reading this chapter and completing the review questions, the reader should be able to:

- Define five possible responsibilities of a marketing manager.
- Describe the role of a director of professional relations.
- List three possible management careers for dental hygienists in the oral healthcare products industry.

Upon graduation from dental hygiene school, my vista was to help humankind prevent periodontal disease! Little did I know that the astute comments of my biology professor from college would lead me to the career I am presently enjoying.

You have read many chapters on different aspects of management and how you might incorporate those business practices in oral healthcare delivery. Working with a manufacturing company challenges you to incorporate your dental hygiene experience within a business/marketing setting. Consider, as an example, a management position in which you would be responsible for marketing an oral health related-product or process to healthcare professionals and/or consumers.

How many dental hygienists work in the oral healthcare products industry or related industries? If asked that question 17 years ago when I embarked on my present career, I would have answered merely a handful. Today it is a different story. Many companies have followed the example of Teledyne Water Pik when, in 1976, it was one of the first companies to utilize dental hygienists to market an oral healthcare product.

**221**

How does one go about getting a job in the oral healthcare products industry? Is it necessary to obtain an advanced degree or have specific experience? No, but you must be alert and in touch with related fields. Be aware of what is going on (i.e., new products, new trends, regulations, opportunities for improvement) and establish a network of peers that will help keep you informed, and inform others of you.

## BACKGROUND

As an example, let me describe how my career has evolved. Hopefully, this will provide some insight into and incentive for you to expand your dental hygiene career into a management role.

When I started in college, I was enrolled in a two-year liberal arts program. As I mentioned, I had a very astute biology professor who recognized my interest in science and encouraged me to think about a career path and suggested research. To make a long story short, I chose dental hygiene for my second two years, thinking I would always have a job that I could rely on and maybe someday could pursue my interest in clinical research and microbiology. Private practice was wonderful, but I wanted more. I was living in a large city but lacked contacts at the universities there, so I started to network to meet people and to find the "who's who list" in the dental research world. I was able to set up an appointment with one of the top researchers at the Forsyth Dental Research Center and had the opportunity to sell myself. When I look back, I wonder why he ever saw me, or how I had the strength to walk in knowing nothing about dental research. Unbeknownst to me, my timing was perfect because Dr. Lobene had just been awarded a National Institutes of Health (NIH) grant and needed a hygienist to work with him on the clinical research project. Thus I was launched on a new career path without a special degree or specific experience—just some good networking.

Two years later I moved to St. Louis and assumed that my new research career was going to be put on hold for a while. I took the regional boards and continued to pursue a job in private practice via the Sunday paper. Blessings continued to follow me. In the paper's classified section, under dental hygiene, ran an advertisement that read "dental hygienist—research background preferred." I was in shock. There were no major universities with ongoing dental research programs (I had already checked for those). Who needed a hygienist with a research background? It was a large chemical company, the Monsanto Corporation, that was embarking on a project to find a better occlusal sealant. I was overwhelmed to find such an opportunity, and at the same time, I realized I had also been shortsighted in my job search because I had not looked past the paradigm with which I was familiar.

The job was a challenge in many ways. I was considered the on-site dental expert, and I worked very closely with the chemists and physicists in the laboratory to develop a new product. Continuous in vitro testing was necessary for plaque growth and adherence. Extracted teeth, which I obtained from dental offices, were used to ensure more realistic testing. After 18 months of laboratory work, we were ready for in vivo testing. Rats are used in caries research because their diets and environments can be controlled. Now I ask you, in all those days in clinic, did you ever in your wildest dreams think that you might be asked one day to clean a rat's teeth? Well, I didn't, but there I was the dental expert! The biggest challenge was to find instruments small enough to fit into their mouths (ophthalmic surgical instruments) in order to apply the sealants properly.

Unfortunately, the project itself was not a success, but the experience was a success for me personally. Six years later, we had done everything from testing toothpaste abrasivity (Monsanto produced a large quantity of phosphates) to plaque adherence with certain cereals. But then the job was cut back to just three days a week, and I began to grow restless. I turned to the Sunday paper. Within six months I was again surprised to find an advertisement that led to my present employment with Teledyne Water Pik. If anyone at that time had told me that I would still be employed by the same company 17 years later, I would have laughed. The advertisement was for a dental hygienist, part-time, who wanted to travel and learn to present product-specific clinical research to dental and dental hygiene schools. I was very fortunate to be chosen for the job, and went on to manage the southeast territory for ten years, during which time I also returned to private practice.

## MANAGING MARKETING

After ten years as a part-time educational consultant, I was offered the opportunity to come "inside" to a full-time position as a professional marketing manager. I really didn't know what a marketing manager was supposed to do, but I knew a great deal about dentistry and dental hygiene, and I thought I was certainly capable of learning the rest.

I am often asked, "As a marketing manager what types of projects are you involved in?" Let me answer this by using my former job responsibilities as examples.

The first thing you must learn to do is plan, and plan responsibly. But before you begin planning, it is essential to have an in-depth understanding of your customer(s) and their wants and needs. A company like Teledyne Water Pik relies on the retail trade to sell their products, yet 70% of those sales are based on professional recommendations. The needs of the two groups are so different, and the information is so diverse, that Teledyne employs two different marketing managers: One works with the trade/retail customers, the other works with the professional customers. As a professional marketing manager, I decided what product information was most pertinent to the professionals and considered what their needs were in educating their patients. Having had no formal marketing training, I was a little overwhelmed the first time my manager asked me to write a marketing plan. Much of the process, though, is a combination of good background knowledge and common sense.

Consider an analogous situation that we all have faced. Imagine you are about to decorate your home. You start with a plan in your mind about how you want it to look. You set up a budget, and then you start to search for pieces that will work together and provide you with the overall look you desire. As you become more familiar with what is available, you may realize that you cannot do it all within the allotted time and budget. You must then begin to prioritize and make difficult choices, some harder than others because the final result is uncertain. What is your alternative at that point? Test a few ideas out, try a few samples, and see how things look.

The same type of process applies to writing a marketing plan and choosing marketing programs that will be effective. As the expert, it was my responsibility to choose the programs that would best accomplish our mission and increase the professional recommendations of our products. It was difficult to know what would be the most effective programs, but I relied on my intuition and tested a few ideas.

You are familiar with professional journal advertisements, direct mail, patient education materials, videos, clinical research supplements, and continuing education courses. Have you ever thought about who develops those materials, and how they decide what content they should include? Think about that the next time you flip through a journal or receive mail in the office. See whether you can tell what companies may have dental hygienists on staff developing the information, and take the time to think about what it took to develop the piece and what you might do differently.

Although it may appear to be simple to write copy, some of the hidden challenges are the restraints imposed by government, trade, and professional organizations. You must follow specific guidelines both with professional and consumer materials to avoid misleading the customer. The American Dental Association, the one organization that truly scrutinizes copy for valid content, has a voluntary evaluation program, and a company chooses whether or not to become involved. The downside for marketing is the restrictions imposed and the time it takes for a review by the scientific board. These delays can have a significant impact in the introduction of a product, service, or feature that is time critical, if you are only a few months or weeks ahead of your competition in reaching your market.

As you are reading this, you may be thinking there is no way that you could accomplish these responsibilities, but think of what you do in private practice. You develop a treatment plan for the client, you set a time frame, you have checkpoints along the way, and you have a budget. You are really more prepared and experienced than you might realize.

Another major responsibility of a marketing manager is to bring visibility to the company within the professional arena, and to promote the quality and leadership that exists within the company and the quality of its products. This is not a difficult task for me while working with Teledyne Water Pik. But again, you learn by trial and error what support programs work toward building a quid pro quo relationship. They may be as simple as developing a much-needed educational grant at a dental or dental hygiene school, or planning a symposium in a rural area, or working with a partner (such as a professional organization) that does not have the funds to conduct or complete a project. I found this a very exciting and challenging part of my job, and I realized that I was relying on tried-and-true dental hygiene–client relationship skills. The more I became involved with it, the more I realized there was nothing magical about building good relationships. You just have to work for a company that you are very proud to represent, and always keep in mind the other person's needs as well as your own. Then you have it made! Actually, I was able to establish such strong relations with people who had a direct contribution or influence on our business that I was promoted to my present position of director of professional relations.

# PROFESSIONAL RELATIONS

With this new title came a whole new set of responsibilities. Allow me to again describe my responsibilities using examples of the management principles that have been previously discussed.

One of the most challenging aspects of the director of professional relations position is the management of people. Teledyne Water Pik is very committed to the Deming philosophy. W. Edwards Deming (1986) was responsible for the post–World War II explosion of the Japanese market and quality product development. Deming teaches that your employees are your most important asset and that all employees want to do a good job—they just need to be led and managed. I have seven people reporting to me at this time. One is my invaluable coordinator, who makes me look good and keeps the ship running smoothly; the other six are dental hygienists responsible for managing their respective territories. These women have all come from backgrounds similar to yours and mine and have chosen to use their dental hygiene experience in an alternative setting.

The director of professional relations is responsible for planning and developing, with the hygienists' valuable input, the programs that the professional department will achieve each year. The hygienists' main function is to disseminate product-specific information and the clinical research to substantiate that product positioning to professionals. This may happen in many different settings, such as dental or dental hygiene school presentations, lectures to national, state, or local continuing education meetings, and dental/dental hygiene conventions. Because of the longevity of this program and the credibility that has been established, there are many days when our time is spent just prioritizing presentations. Remembering back to the development of a plan, there is also a timetable to be followed and a budget to be managed. This generates a lot of administrative paperwork for a program like this, which has to be managed on a day-to-day basis.

The director of professional relations also manages both the domestic and European advisory boards; which consist of extremely influential and knowledgeable thought and opinion leaders. In this position, it is important that I take the time to establish my own trustworthiness and credibility so that a comfortable exchange of information may take place. Both individual consultants and boards are utilized for development of pertinent clinical research projects and new products and as a reality check on many of our marketing programs.

The advisory boards usually meet at least once or twice a year at various locations. (Not too long ago I had to "suffer" through a meeting in a castle in Kronberg, Germany!) Although I do my best to plan for the consulting time of the advisers, there are possibilities of unanticipated events that may present unique opportunities. As these arise, we may review the budget and reprioritize our anticipated expenses to take advantage of the opportunity. One thing you quickly learn in industry: there is not an endless supply of money. Your advertising and sales promotion moneys are a direct percentage of your sales.

Another of my functions is to serve as liaison between professional organizations and the company. Some of the organizations that Teledyne Water Pik works with are the American Academy of Periodontology, the American Dental Hygienists' Association, the American Dental Association, the American Fund for Dental

Health, and the Academy of General Dentistry. Of all of these associations, the American Dental Association is probably the most challenging. Back in the beginning of this chapter, when I was describing the responsibilities of a marketing manager, I made reference to some difficulties in regard to development of advertising copy with imposed regulations. Let me expand on that point as I elaborate on my liaison duties.

If a manufacturer of a dental product desires to carry the ADA logo and seal of approval on its package, it must voluntarily submit all marketing materials to the ADA board of review for approval before publication. Think of the implications. If you decide that the ADA seal is important to your customers, and you have solid substantiation of your claims to earn the seal but some of your competitors do not, they cannot carry the seal, but they can make just about any claim they want with no accountability. At times it is frustrating, but our customers continue to tell us it is important to see the ADA logo. Therefore my job is to facilitate the submission and review of copy to the ADA and to have as quick a turn-around time as possible. Also, to keep communication as open and as clear as possible, I am usually the sole contact with the ADA for any other projects we are working on.

## Summary

I hope that you come away from reading this chapter realizing that many new and exciting opportunities are developing for dental hygienists. Do not limit yourself to your existing frame, but rather think about a new paradigm and what it might take to work in it. The fact that you have picked up this book is a great indication that you want more. Do not be afraid of it; explore your options. What is the worst that can happen? One door may close, but usually another one will open.

## Review Questions

1. Define five possible responsibilities of a marketing manager.
2. Describe the role of a director of professional relations.
3. List three possible management careers for dental hygienists in the oral health-care products industry.
4. Choose a product that you find interesting. Based on the content of advertisements, direct mail, consumer materials, information gathered at meetings, and any other available sources, describe what you think the manufacturer's marketing plan (price, position, promotion) is for the product.
5. Create your own marketing plan for the product you investigated in Question 4.
6. Describe ways in which your marketing plan differs from the manufacturer's plan you described in Question 4.

7. Describe the challenges and opportunities you think you might find in managing a team of educational representatives.

8. Write a marketing plan for marketing yourself as a manager to an oral healthcare products firm like Teledyne Water Pik.

## SUGGESTED READING

Mackey, H. (1988). *Swim with the sharks without being eaten alive.* New York: William Morrow & Co.

Von Oech, R. (1990). *A whack on the side of the head.* New York: Warner Books.

Williamson, J. N. (1986). *The leader manager.* New York: John Wiley & Sons.

## REFERENCE

Deming, W. E. (1986). *Out of the crisis.* Cambridge, Mass.: MIT, Center for Advanced Engineering Study.

CHAPTER 13

# Public Health

## *Objectives*

After reading this chapter and completing the review questions, the reader should be able to:

- Discuss career opportunities within public health programs for dental hygienists, noting the associated education and skills needed.

- Write a mission statement, goals, objectives, action plans, timelines, and evaluation methods for a dental public health program.

- Discuss factors in public-supported agencies that impact on an administrator's ability to manage programs, personnel, and budget.

- Describe the importance of oral health needs assessment and community needs assessment for program planning, resource allocation, and evaluation.

- Discuss limitations in public health programs related to marketing, advocacy, and lobbying, and avenues for overcoming these problems.

- Outline resources available at local, state, regional, and national levels to assist managers of dental public health programs.

- Discuss the concepts of leadership and vision as they apply to management skills and public health programs.

- Give examples of issues in public health agencies that relate to management of personnel.

- Outline important questions to ask when interviewing for a management position in dental public health and during orientation to the new position.

- Describe a dental public health manager's role in developing policies, procedures, rules and regulations, and legislative testimony.

# THE FIELD OF DENTAL PUBLIC HEALTH

The definition of "dental public health" as developed by the American Board of Public Health and approved by public health organizations states:

> Dental public health is the science and art of preventing and controlling dental diseases and promoting dental health through organized community efforts. It is that form of dental practice which serves the community as a patient rather than the individual. It is concerned with the dental education of the public, with applied dental research, and with the administration of group dental care programs as well as the prevention and control of dental diseases on a community basis. [Burt & Eklund, 1992]

The field of dental public health is so diverse in terms of employment settings and job responsibilities that a single chapter cannot begin to provide a comprehensive review of management aspects. I have chosen therefore to share insights and examples from my own public health experiences to highlight some of the issues I feel are important for a dental hygienist who chooses a career in public health.

Many people share the misconception that dental hygienists who work in the public health arena are merely providing clinical dental hygiene services to clients who receive care in government-supported programs. In truth, most public health hygienists function on an entirely different level and do not focus the majority of their efforts on individual client care. Much of their job involves program development, coordination, and evaluation for subgroups of the public or specific projects. Therefore their mindset in terms of mission, goals, objectives, and activities differs from that of clinical hygienists. Also, they may have to relate to a whole network of agencies, other professionals, financing mechanisms, and rules and regulations—foreign territory to most private practitioners.

# JOB OPPORTUNITIES AND CAREERS

What are some public health programs or settings where dental hygienists might seek employment or consulting opportunities? The following examples provide an overview of positions held by hygienists. Job availability and job responsibilities may vary by agency and geographic location.

- Consultant to the World Health Organization on dental hygiene personnel needed in Third World countries
- Health promotion/disease prevention coordinator for a regional office of the Indian Health Service
- Commissioned officer providing clinical care and training at a naval training program
- Dental hygiene program coordinator for a federal correctional facility
- Dental hygienist for a Veterans' Administration medical center with an affiliated geriatric education center
- Branch chief in the division of oral health at the Centers for Disease Control and Prevention

- Consultant on OSHA compliance and infection control
- Professor in a community dentistry department of a dental school or dental hygiene program
- State dental director in a state health department
- Program coordinator for oral health in a maternal and child health program in a state department of child and family services
- Public health adviser in the Radiologic and Medical Devices Division of the Federal Drug Administration
- Research analyst for the Health Resources and Services Administration
- Oral epidemiologist at the National Institute for Dental Research
- Public health educator in a county health department
- Coordinator of school-based projects for a nonprofit community dental health agency
- Dental hygiene coordinator for a mobile dental health project for homebound and institutionalized elders
- Site coordinator for the National Health Interview Survey
- Dental hygienist for a summer migrant health program
- Dental health manager of a multiagency dental program for the homeless
- Head Start dental health consultant

You can see the variety of opportunities in the titles, agencies, and population groups represented in these examples. This variety is what makes public health jobs challenging and enables us to develop skills that we may not have learned during our dental hygiene education. Most hygienists who work in public health have sought additional education, earning their baccalaureate, master's, or doctoral degrees in fields such as public health, health administration, health education, gerontology, community health, business administration, or public policy. Others have developed additional skills through continuing education courses, fellowships, internships, on-the-job training, volunteer opportunities, and self-directed readings or writing for publication. Most administrative positions now require at least a master's degree. As you read this chapter, think about the specific skills dental public health managers need and ways you might start to acquire some of them.

To familiarize you with public-supported employment opportunities, let's look at some general employment trends in federal, state, and local governments.

## Trends in Federal Employment

Federal employment via the civil service system has remained a fairly stable career option over the past 20 to 30 years, although significant fluctuations may occur across or within agencies. This makes a manager's job in federal agencies somewhat difficult yet challenging because you're never sure whether you'll be dealing with an expanding or shrinking work force and budget. Also, with political appointments, changes occur with every administration and Congress.

In terms of geography, the mid-Atlantic and southeastern areas of the United States are home to about one-third of all federal employees. This does depend on the agency and specific programs, however. For example, most Indian Health Service positions are located in the western regions of the United States, while Veterans' Administration programs are distributed across the country.

About 25% of federal jobs are professional, technical, or management related; this percentage is projected to increase by the year 2000 (Johnson et al., 1988). Dental hygienists usually would apply for jobs in these categories. Management related means that you don't have to supervise others directly, but you do provide staff and support services such as program analysis or training. There are separate classifications for supervisory and nonsupervisory positions. Job classifications are not necessarily comparable to the dental titles we would encounter in other settings. For instance, dental hygienists could apply for job categories such as education specialist, public health adviser, public health educator, technical writer, or project manager. These positions may or may not require a dental hygiene background, degree, or license, but may instead look at particular skills you possess. Career ladders specifically for dental hygienists in the federal system are extremely limited and many clinical positions are still at very low pay scales. Employee benefits and opportunities for continuing education and travel are fairly generous, however. Other trends predicted for employment in the federal civil service system include (Burt & Eklund, 1992):

- The average age of the federal work force will rise; the median age is about 36 today.
- More women and minorities will enter the work force.
- Positions will require higher skill levels and educational attainment.
- Public esteem and prestige of government jobs will decline.
- Long-term stability will decline in some agencies.
- Agencies will be more dependent on Congress for budget.
- Competition from the private sector will increase for highly qualified people.

Recently there has been a trend to contract out for services as a way to downsize the permanent government work force and rebuild private enterprise and small businesses. This may be an avenue for dental hygienists who want to be contractors to become involved in federal programs; note that employee benefits such as insurance and vacation are not provided to contractors. Another avenue recently opened to qualified hygienists is to join the Commissioned Corps—a uniformed arm of the Public Health Service. This career is an alternative to the civil service system for those who qualify and are considering a career in the Public Health Service. Applicants have to possess at least a baccalaureate degree and be under age 44. Pay scales and benefits tend to be more liberal than in the civil service system.

The three career avenues just described—civil service, private contracting, and commissioned corps—really refer only to employment/personnel systems or arrangements. Job opportunities and responsibilities are similar across these systems and will vary by agency, locale, and focus of the programs.

## Trends in State Employment

State governments expanded during the 1980s but the recent economic downturn has caused state legislatures and governors to balance budgets by downsizing the government work force and eliminating programs. As layoffs increase in both the private and public sectors, more people become eligible for entitlement programs such as Medicaid. Such programs then consume more of the budget, thus threatening other health programs. Dental programs have been fairly hard hit during this process, with some states eliminating state dental director positions or entire programs. Others are conducting innovative programs with few resources. In some instances this has created greater opportunities for dental hygienists as health promotion programs replace direct care programs or as dentists' salaries become unaffordable. Since dollars earmarked directly for dental programs are becoming scarce, programs that incorporate an interdisciplinary approach (such as AIDS or injury control) may tend to prosper. Benefits in state systems are comparable to those in the federal civil service system but recent budget deficits in some states have prompted legislatures to interfere with previously negotiated raises and other benefits such as health insurance.

## City and Local Governments

Employment in this sector is greatly affected by what occurs at the state and federal level. As statewide subsidies for services are eliminated or reduced, local programs are forced to increase their support for some services while eliminating others. The trend to outside contracting and privatization is also occurring at the local level.

To familiarize you with the actual responsibilities of a dental public health manager, let's start by discussing the various aspects of program planning and evaluation, remembering that it is difficult to make generalizations due to the variety of agencies involved in the public health arena.

# PROGRAM MANAGEMENT

Public health programs rely on principles of the planning cycle as described in Chapter 1 for their long-range strategic plans and for their daily activities. In fact, there may be multiple planning cycles that often overlap. For instance, when I was director of a state dental program, we received moneys from a biennial state budget that extended from July 1, 1992, to June 30, 1994. We also received federal moneys based on the federal budget, which spanned from October 1, 1992, to September 30, 1993. Holiday and vacation periods were determined on a calendar year, from January 1 to December 31. Personnel evaluations and raises were based on annual anniversary date of hiring. As a manager, I had the task of planning for and coordinating personnel, budgets, and activities that took into account all of these timelines and factors so that services and employee benefits ran smoothly and without interruption.

The planning process in public health involves multiple layers of managers so that communication and timing across these layers is important but difficult. In many instances, decisions must be made quickly, based on limited data. In other instances, decisions are made that significantly impact your program, whether or not you have had any input into those decisions. These are frustrating aspects of managing public health programs. One frequent mistake, particularly in direct care programs, is for managers and staff to become overwhelmed by daily activities and not devote time to planning and evaluation. Such programs often become stagnant or are eliminated. Managers who devote time to planning will have anticipated potential problems and can mobilize alternative plans.

## Mission Statement

A clear mission statement is critical for dental public health programs since many people do not understand the primary purpose of dental programs except to provide direct dental treatment. Using the previous definition of dental public health, we can expand and update it to create a mission statement for a specific program. For example: "The Division of Oral Health seeks to prevent and control oral diseases and promote oral health of the citizens of the town of Rhineholt through organized community efforts. We conduct dental health education and health promotion campaigns, applied dental research projects, and community-based prevention programs as well as formulate policies and regulations to assure the public's safety and health."

## Goals and Objectives

While the mission statement for a program will probably remain unchanged over a period of time, the goals and objectives may change on an annual basis. Figure 13.1 provides an example of goals and objectives for a federally funded three-state project to identify oral health needs of the elderly population and develop state plans to meet those needs. Note that the expected outcomes also serve as evaluation measures.

Currently, public health programs and federal funding are being driven by the Year 2000 Health Objectives for the Nation (USDHHS, 1991). States have adapted these 16 objectives (see Figure 13.2) and developed action plans to reflect their own program emphases and baseline data.

The Year 2000 objectives are long-range. Program managers can create associated short-term objectives or establish specific targets for data collection to monitor progress. These oral health objectives also emphasize the importance of establishing baseline data for objectives so that a surveillance system can be instituted to track progress. A challenge for dental public health program managers is to plan and find methods for collecting the necessary data and to carry out appropriate activities to meet the objectives. The Centers for Disease Control and Prevention, Division of Oral Health, plays a key role in providing technical assistance to state agencies to facilitate this process.

| Goals | Objectives | Outcomes |
|---|---|---|
| Primary Goal: To improve the oral health of the elderly population. | | |
| Secondary Goals: | | |
| 1. Establish formal linkages between "organized" dentistry and dental hygiene, state AOAs, AHECs, and dental and dental hygiene schools on a statewide basis. | 1.1 Form a steering committee in each of four states with representatives from each of these organizations. | 1.11 Written reports and attendance by at least 85% of the committee. |
| | 1.2 Write letters of agreement for cooperative efforts with each of these organizations. | 1.21 Formal letters of agreement approved by each organization. |
| 2. Increase knowledge of dental and aging network professionals and paraprofessionals about the oral health needs of the elderly and programs and resources to meet those needs. | 2.1 Develop and provide continuing education forums based on identified needs of both healthcare consumers and healthcare providers. | 2.11 Receipt by at least a certain percentage of professionals and paraprofessionals (as pre-determined by each state's steering committee) of continuing education related to oral health needs of the elderly. |
| | 2.2 Disseminate information about the project and oral health needs of the elderly via oral and written mechanisms. | 2.21 Articles and papers presented in at least five newsletters, four journals, and three meetings. |

3. Establish a coordinated statewide and regional approach to long-range planning for addressing the dental needs of the elderly population.

3.1 Conduct regular planning meetings in each state.

3.11 At least three planning meetings during the project period.

3.2 Analyze needs assessment data.

3.21 Descriptions of oral health needs and barriers to care of the elderly in four states.

3.3 Identify resources for meeting the dental needs of the elderly and the continuing education needs of professionals and paraprofessionals in each state.

3.31 List of material and personnel resources for each state for: (a) providing dental care; (b) implementing continuing education programs.

3.4 Develop statewide plan for meeting the identified needs.

3.41 Written state plans for meeting the identified needs in four states (includes who is responsible for each segment).

**Figure 13.1**  *Goals, objectives, and outcomes*

13.1    Reduce dental caries so that the proportion of children with one or more caries in permanent or primary teeth is no more than 35% among children aged 6–8 and no more than 60% among adolescents aged 15. (Baseline: 53% of 6- to 8-year-olds and 78% of 15-year-olds in 1986–1987)

13.2    Reduce untreated dental caries so that the proportion of children with untreated caries in permanent or primary teeth is no more than 20% among children aged 6–8 and no more than 15% among adolescents aged 15. (Baseline: 27% of 6- to 8-year-olds and 23% of 15-year-olds in 1986)

13.3    Increase to at least 45% the proportion of people aged 35–44 who have never lost a permanent tooth due to dental caries or periodontal diseases. (Baseline: 31% of employed adults in 1985–1986)

13.4    Reduce to no more than 20% the proportion of people aged 65 and older who have lost all of their natural teeth. (Baseline: 36% in 1986)

13.5    Reduce the prevalence of gingivitis among people aged 35–44 to no more than 30%. (Baseline: 42% in 1985–1986)

13.6    Reduce destructive periodontal diseases to a prevalence of no more than 15% among people aged 35–44. (Baseline: 24% in 1985–1986)

13.7    Reduce deaths due to cancer of the oral cavity and pharynx to no more than 10.5 per 100,000 men aged 45–74 and 4.1 per 100,000 women aged 45–74. (Baseline: 12.1 per 100,000 men and 4.1 per 100,000 women in 1987)

13.8    Increase to at least 50% the proportion of children who have received protective sealants on the occlusal surfaces of permanent molar teeth. (Baseline: 11% of 8-year-olds and 8% of 14-year-olds in 1986–1987)

13.9    Increase to at least 75% the proportion of people served by community water systems providing optimal levels of fluoride. (Baseline: 62% in 1989)

13.10   Increase use of professionally or self-administered topical or systemic fluorides to at least 85% of people not receiving optimally fluoridated public water. (Baseline: 50% in 1989)

13.11   Increase to at least 75% the proportion of parents and caregivers who use feeding practices that prevent baby bottle tooth decay. (Baseline not yet available)

13.12   Increase to at least 90% the proportion of all children entering school programs for the first time who have received an oral health screening, referral, and follow-up for necessary diagnostic, preventive, and treatment services. (Baseline: 66% of 5-year-olds visited a dentist during 1985)

13.13   Extend to all long-term institutional facilities the requirement that oral examinations and services be provided no later than 90 days after entry into these facilities. (Baseline: data unavailable)

13.14   Increase to at least 70% the proportion of people aged 35 and older using the oral healthcare system during each year. (Baseline: 54% in 1986)

13.15   Increase to at least 40 the number of states that have an effective system for recording and referring infants with cleft lips and/or palates to craniofacial anomaly teams. (Baseline: 25 states)

13.16   Extend requirement of the use of effective head, face, eye, and mouth protection to all organizations, agencies, and institutions sponsoring sporting and recreation events that pose risks of injury. (Baseline: only NCAA football, hockey, and lacrosse; high school football; amateur boxing; amateur ice hockey in 1988)

**Figure 13.2**    *Year 2000 objectives for oral care*

## Target Groups

Decisions to target specific groups for services generally are based on age, income, residence, disability, or disease criteria for eligibility or entitlement. Examples of targeted programs include Head Start, WIC (Women, Infants and Children), Medicaid, Medicare, Meals on Wheels, Hospice, Migrant Health Centers, Nursing Home Mobile Dental Programs, and Ryan White funds for AIDS patients. Generally more people are eligible for programs than funding allows, so multiple targeting approaches based on priorities and extent of needs are necessary. Needs are assessed through a variety of mechanisms.

## Oral Health Program Needs Assessment

When designing dental public health programs you would first try to determine oral health status, perceived needs of the public, attitudes toward prevention and dental care, knowledge of oral diseases and prevention methods, preventive behaviors, barriers to care, manpower availability and expertise, and availability and cost of equipment and supplies. Suggested readings at the end of the chapter provide specific examples of how to obtain this information. All methods differ in regard to cost, complexity, time involvement, and need for human resources. The role of the manager is to select the most valid and cost-effective methods for obtaining and analyzing the desired information. Unfortunately, skills in needs assessment still seem to be a weak component in most hygienists' education.

The needs assessment process should involve members and opinion leaders of potential target groups, program staff of related programs, and potential providers of care. Focus groups, individual interviews, "town hall" meetings, health boards, or advisory groups are a few examples of ways to gain input. The manager must summarize and analyze this advice (which often represents conflicting viewpoints), consider it in light of the oral health status data, and mold it into program priorities and activities that can be evaluated. This process relates directly to the total quality management principles described in previous chapters. Figure 13.3 demonstrates a short case study of the needs assessment process and links the findings to program outcomes.

An equally important step in a needs assessment, but one that sometimes is forgotten, is to create a written summary of the information, documenting why particular groups are targeted or justifying activities selected. Some form of this report should be disseminated back to people who participated in the needs assessment so they can see how their input was used. This step will not necessarily create advocates for your program, but it may reduce the number of vocal adversaries, start dialog with diverse interest groups, and educate people about the diverse needs of a community.

## Advocacy

The issue of advocacy is extremely important to public and nonprofit programs, since program continuation depends on how it is perceived by people other than you or your staff. The primary way to create internal advocacy or marketing is to

**Request**

The Lewis City Homeless Project asked the County Dental Health Division to assess the dental health needs of homeless persons in the city to determine whether funds for dental care should be included in the budget.

**Planning**

Because of staff shortages and budget reductions, the county dental director met with faculty at a nearby dental school to enlist the help of two students to perform interviews and an oral health survey. Supplies were to be provided by the Dental Division. A faculty member also agreed to assist the dental director in designing the study, printing the survey forms, and analyzing the data. Two shelter programs were chosen as survey sites: The Lloyd Center, serving primarily single males; and the Sonis House, serving singles and families with children. One staff member at each shelter was assigned to coordinate schedules and enlist volunteers.

**Survey**

One hundred adults completed written questionnaires/oral interviews and an oral inspection. Measures of oral health status looked at number of teeth, dental caries, periodontal disease, and need for care. Participants answered questions about perceived dental needs, past use of care, opinions about what services should be available, preventive health behaviors, and risk factors for oral problems.

**Survey Results**

Analysis of data revealed that 60% of the people were "recently homeless" and had received some care in the past. Twenty percent needed immediate care for infections or toothaches, while 20% had no obvious needs. The majority needed basic restorative care, periodontal therapy, and improved oral hygiene practices. Most also needed a new toothbrush with a protective cover and toothpaste. Dental care was ranked high on a list of health services they felt were needed.

**Presentation to the Homeless Project Board**

A poster display of the data was used to present the information to the Board. Handouts were also provided. All materials were left with the Board to share with shelter staff and participants. The director of the Dental Health Division and the dental students who participated led the discussion.

**Outcomes**

As a result of the needs assessment, the Board voted to include a request for dental care in its budget as a special initiative. It also developed a Cooperative Agreement with the Division of Dental Health and the Dental School to design a dental program that could be used as a training site for dental and dental hygiene students under the supervision of a clinic director. Emergency and preventive procedures would be priorities for care, especially for homeless families. Social services staff for the shelters would be responsible for scheduling appointments. Prior to the opening of the on-site clinic, homeless persons would be seen at the Dental School and the Division of Dental Health would provide toothbrushes and toothpaste to the shelters.

**Figure 13.3** *Needs assessment case study*

publicize the benefits and program effectiveness through various media or reports. For long-term involvement, building coalitions with other individuals or organizations, particularly members of the target groups that receive services, is more effective. This is extremely important when the program is being considered for continuation or budget reductions by the legislature or by a governing board. Professional organizations, private businesses, and agencies that are amenable to cooperative projects are strong allies.

Unfortunately, decisions for funding often are made by people who know little about the program and who only listen to taxpayers who may not be recipients of these services. Government employees are not allowed to lobby for their programs with legislators so it is imperative that dental public health programs have strong supporters in the community who can contact these people. Elected officials generally listen to their constituents more than to agency staff, no matter what level of government they serve.

To market a program, the manager must be a timely disseminator of information in a format that the general public will understand. Writing in such a format is an interesting task for professionals who are used to dealing with technical and scientific terms. Asking nondental people to review such information before it is disseminated is advisable. Figure 13.4 provides an example of how one program "translated" technical program information for the public and attempted to create a forum for exchange of information.

Advocacy for oral health programs at a national level primarily is spearheaded by the Oral Health Section of the American Public Health Association, the American Association of Public Health Dentistry, the Association of State and Territorial Dental Directors, the Association of Community Dental Programs, the Division of Oral Health in the Centers for Disease Control and Prevention, and staff in the various agencies of the U.S. Department of Health and Human Services. These groups form coalitions with other dental and nondental groups to promote initiatives such as the Year 2000 Objectives and inclusion of oral health in National Health Care Reform. Membership in professional public health organizations and regular contact with public health staff in federal or state programs is crucial for any manager of a dental public health program.

## Matching Resources to Services

The source and stipulations attached to moneys that support dental public health programs influence the focus of those programs. Two major federal funding sources for statewide public health programs, the Maternal and Child Health Block Grant and the Preventive Health and Health Services Block Grant, include specific program foci but allow a great deal of flexibility in the variety of services provided and the subgroups targeted. Some state health departments use these funds specifically for direct dental care services and school-based fluoride supplement programs. Other states fund fluoride tablet programs for Well Child Clinics, health promotion programs for a variety of ages, and training workshops for other health providers.

The focus of any particular program also depends on the results of needs assessments, community resources available, and the number and type of staff employed

---

**Exhibit A (Technical Version)**

**Oral Cancer Epidemiology, Risk Factors, and Symptoms**
More than 1 million Americans will develop cancers each year. About 30,000 of
these will be oral and oropharyngeal cancers. The five-year survival rate is only
about 35%. When diagnosed, 50% of these cancers will already have
metastasized. Stage 1 and 2 oral cancers may be painless or asymptomatic.
Predisposing factors include chronic irritation of the oral mucosa, repeated
trauma, overexposure to ultraviolet radiation, chronic inflammatory conditions
due to nutritional disorders, alcoholism, and certain viruses. Early signs of
malignancies or premalignancies include erythroplasia or leukoplakia. Late
signs include nodal enlargement and ulcerations.

**Exhibit B (Version for the General Public)**

**What You Should Know About Oral Cancer**
Each year about 3 percent of Americans (30,000 people) develop cancers of the
mouth. More than 60 percent of these people will die within 5 years.
Unfortunately, most people already have advanced stages of disease by the time
they are diagnosed because they don't feel any pain or see any symptoms.
    What things can lead to oral cancers?

- use of tobacco, especially chewing tobacco
- heavy drinking of alcohol
- sharp edges of dentures that create sores that don't heal
- excessive sunlight on the lips
- certain nutritional problems
- some types of viruses

Be aware of these signs and symptoms.

- red or white spots or sores that don't heal
- sores that crack or bleed
- swellings or lumps in the neck or in the mouth

Do you want to learn more about ways to prevent oral cancer?

Come visit our display and meet the dental staff during the Wellness Fair at the
Health Clinic on April 15.

**Figure 13.4**    *Translating technical information to the public*

---

to administer or implement services. States with strong county or local health
departments with established dental clinics may tend to use more resources on
direct dental treatment while states with no local health department infrastructure
and state agency staff with strong health promotion backgrounds will probably
focus resources on health promotion activities. Management responsibilities and
skills will be very different for each of these programs. Hygienists who try to
become managers in states with strong restorative care dental programs and strong
state dental associations may find their jobs much more limited than hygienists who
move into positions that do not require the clinical or technical expertise of a dentist. Again, this will depend on how the programs are set up and on the role of the

1. What are the self-perceived strengths, interests, and areas for improvement for each staff member?
2. What do you perceive as their strengths and areas for improvement?
3. What additional skills do they want to learn? How can these skills be acquired? Mentoring? Agency-sponsored workshops? College courses? Who provides the funding?
4. What opportunities are available for staff to use these skills once they are learned?
5. What skills do you need from the staff to run the program effectively?
6. Do current staff have these skills or can they learn them? If not, do you need additional staff with different skills?
7. Will you be allowed to hire additional staff with different skills? If not, how will you have to change services to fit the skill levels of your staff?
8. How much of your time as an administrator is consumed performing program tasks because of staff shortages or inadequate staff skills?

**Figure 13.5**   *Assessing staffing needs and abilities of staff*

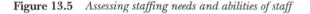

manager in relation to the clinical programs. Many hygienists are excellent managers of public and nonprofit direct care dental programs. They have sufficient clinical staff to implement clinical services and provide direct supervision for their programs. Unfortunately, many people confuse "management and administrative skills" with "clinical and professional supervision requirements" outlined in state practice acts, thus restricting some management positions to dentists.

Along with doing a community needs assessment, managers should assess the needs and abilities of their staff. Figure 13.5 offers pertinent questions that may help managers in this process. The answers to these questions may be affected by the downsizing occurring in many agencies and businesses. Clients expect the same level of services or expanded services, yet managers are being asked to provide "more with less." Managers in these situations must be able to communicate "reality" to consumers and higher-level administrators so that expectations are realistic yet the quality of services is not compromised and staff are not demoralized. If expectations remain unrealistic, then the manager and staff are in untenable positions that quickly lead to burnout.

Up to this stage in the planning process, we have been discussing issues related to initial stages of program planning, specifically, development of a mission statement, conducting needs assessments, and writing goals and objectives. Let's continue with the planning process and assume that staff issues have been addressed. From goals and objectives, action plans and timelines need to be formulated.

## Creating Action Plans and Timelines

Figure 13.6 displays tasks and timelines for the project outlined in Figure 13.1. Notice that some tasks require only a short period of time to accomplish, while others are ongoing over many months. In this example, tasks are listed sequentially as they would occur, with some happening simultaneously. A timeline for a

Month

| Task | 1 | 2 | 3 | 4 | 5 | 6 | 7 | 8 | 9 | 10 | 11 | 12 | 13 | 14 | 15 | 16 | 17 |
|---|---|---|---|---|---|---|---|---|---|---|---|---|---|---|---|---|---|
| 1. States assign project reps | ↕ | ↕ | | | | | | | | | | | | | | | |
| 2. Develop needs assessment | | ↕ | ↕ | | | | | | | | | | | | | | |
| 3. States collect preliminary needs assessment data | | | | ↕ | | | | ↕ | | | | | | | | | |
| 4. Arrange first meeting in each state | | | ↕ | ↕ | | | | | | | | | | | | | |
| 5. Develop preliminary list of resources | | ↕ | | | ↕ | | | | | | | | | | | | |
| 6. Conduct first steering committee meeting in each state | | | | | ↕ | ↕ | | | | | | | | | | | |
| 7. Plan CE and care activities | | | | | | | | | ↕ | | ↕ | | | | | | |
| 8. Conduct CE and care activities | | | | | | | | | | | | | ↕ | | ↕ | | |
| 9. Conduct second steering committee meeting and finalize state plan | | | | | | | | ↕ | ↕ | | | | | | | | |
| 10. Disseminate project information | | | | | | | | | | ↕ | | ↕ | | | | | |
| 11. Write final report | | | | | | | | | | | | | | | | ↕ | ↕ |

**Figure 13.6** *Tasks and timelines*

particular task is usually displayed as a range of time (e.g., one to two weeks), since so many variables impact on schedules. This allows for some flexibility in the implementation process. As tasks and timelines are developed, names of the staff responsible should be inserted so that assignments are clear and work loads can be distributed equitably.

## Evaluating Outcomes

As mentioned previously, evaluation mechanisms need to be designed as you develop your goals, objectives, and action plans. One of the problems observed in many public health programs is lack of an evaluation plan. If a program is limited to activities such as conducting sealant programs, school mouth rinse sessions, health fairs, library story hours, and in-service training sessions for nursing home staff, the purpose of the activity may be lost. The ultimate goal—the desired outcome—from any of these activities is improved oral health, yet what do we usually measure? Knowledge levels, compliance, number of participants, and number of materials distributed. Why? They are short-term effects that can be "counted." Documenting improved oral health requires that we know the original oral health status (baseline data) and that we measure oral health again sometime in the future. Since most oral diseases take a long time to develop, reducing dental disease or improving oral health status is a long-term process and often costly. While it may be simpler to assume that what we're doing is effective because we were taught about these activities in school, scientific knowledge advances. What we know about dental caries, fluorides, periodontal diseases, and oral cancers today is somewhat different, and the disease patterns are different. Managers must always keep the issue of evaluation in the forefront, especially when documenting effectiveness and accounting for how funds are spent. Quality assurance programs are an integral component in any public health program.

This concludes the section on program planning and evaluation. Let's proceed to a discussion of some personal characteristics that are useful for managers.

# LEADERSHIP AND VISION

Previous chapters outlined the differences among management, leadership, and vision. Although management skills often are taught in educational programs, leadership skills are more difficult to acquire, and vision is an amorphous characteristic that comes easily to some and never to others. Burt Nanus (1992) defines vision as a "realistic, credible, attractive future for your organization." A visionary person inspires action and helps to shape the future through four major roles: direction setter, change agent, spokesperson, and coach. Some people feel that the field of dental public health has suffered from lack of leadership and vision in recent years, so some programs intentionally are looking for these qualities in new administrators. Interviewers may even ask pointed questions about your leadership or management style and what your vision is for the program.

In the public health setting, managers need to be flexible, respond to local needs, keep abreast of national trends, and comply with federal mandates. The visionary manager uses his ability to listen, synthesize, integrate, and reflect about aspects of program objectives. This role requires confidence, a willingness to take risks and take responsibility for actions, and an understanding of dental public health's relationship to other public health programs.

Communication among staff and across programs is essential in any program. Although most dental public health programs are physically located with other types of health programs, this does not ensure open communication. Most people don't understand the range of activities that can occur in dental public health programs. Education is a major responsibility of a manager. Dental public health managers need to be assertive and explain programs and ways in which they can be integrated with other programs. It is a mistake to wait to be invited to participate in activities. We need to create the opportunities.

In 1974 a group of dental public health professionals compiled a document, "Behavioral Objectives for Dental Public Health," to define the competency base for the field (Hughes, 1978). These objectives were rewritten in 1988 at a national workshop, and the resulting document published in 1990 ("Competency Objectives," 1990). This is an excellent reference document for dental public health managers, since 39 of the objectives specifically address health policy, program management, and administration.

A couple of other references also may be useful. "Thirteen Fatal Errors Managers Make and How You Can Avoid Them" (Brown, 1985) provides a useful list with accompanying narrative. My favorites in his list are:

- Refuse to accept personal accountability.
- Fail to develop people.
- Try to control results instead of influencing thinking.
- Fail to set standards.

In Quick's book (1990), "Unconventional Wisdom, Irreverent Solutions for Tough Problems at Work," two survival points particularly apply to the field of public health:

1. You need to become comfortable with ambiguity.
2. The essence of humor is incongruity.

## PERSONNEL MANAGEMENT

Managing people in public health programs is probably one of the most challenging aspects of program administration. In a small private business that is nonunionized, you truly are "the boss" and employees are accountable to you. Employees in a public health program theoretically are accountable to the "public," although managers are still supervisors. Layers of bureaucracy, rules, policies, and union negotiations can influence the way this supervisory role is carried out.

Recruitment and hiring of staff can be a long-term process that involves affirmative action policies; regulations on how, when, and where jobs are advertised; standard interviewing procedures sometimes preceded by "panel" selection based on a written test or oral board; considerations for Native American, veteran, or other minority preference; and specific documentation on why each candidate was or was not selected. To confound the situation, at any time in the process, hiring freezes can be imposed during times of budget deficits.

Although personnel systems in public-supported programs are designed to prevent hiring and promotional biases and abuses and to "manage risk," the complexity of the systems may create a manager's nightmare, especially if a new manager is inadequately oriented to the personnel system. Civil service point systems for "time in grade" and specific classifications of positions become extremely important issues during periods of layoffs or promotions, since employees may be able to "bump" into someone else's job based on seniority, or lose seniority points if they get promoted to a higher-level position. These situations create havoc for program planning, continuity, career development, and employee morale. As a manager, I often have been put in the difficult position of trying to balance decisions that are best for the program with those that are best for the personal survival or professional growth of individual employees.

One mechanism I use to enhance employee morale is to ask everyone to develop a set of personal growth objectives along with professional performance objectives for the year. This allows each person to identify interests, strengths, and areas for improvement. As a manager in a system that was devastated by a severe economic crisis, there was no mechanism for rewarding staff through merit increases or automatic promotions. Instead, I chose to facilitate development of people's skills so they could improve their self-esteem and learn skills that could be translated to other aspects of their lives or to other jobs. The reward of watching demoralized staff bloom into self-confident professionals with balanced personal lives has maintained my enthusiasm and belief in the benefits of a career in management.

Although some of my statements may be construed as negative, they are not meant to dissuade hygienists from becoming managers in governmental programs. They are simply reality statements from my experiences and reflect situations for which educational programs did not prepare me. In most cases we learn to manage these situations on the job and there may not be any "right" answers or guidelines. Figure 13.7 displays a list of questions for new managers that may help when interviewing for or beginning a new position in a public health agency. Some of the questions should be asked when interviewing for a job to determine whether the job meets your expectations and is a good fit. The information allows you to make an informed decision about settings in which you would be unhappy or unable to meet your personal and professional goals. Other questions relate to the orientation process. Finding answers to these questions and posing "what if" questions at the outset will save valuable time and avoid potentially devastating future mistakes. Orientation programs for managers often are in place on paper, but functionally don't exist. Once you begin a new position, find yourself a good mentor who has worked in the agency long enough to know "who to go to for what." Many times this will be administrative staff, not the director.

## Other Administrative Responsibilities

A few responsibilities are unique to public health programs in governmental agencies. Government is responsible for policy development, passage of laws, and pro-

1. Is there an up-to-date organizational chart you can review?

2. Who is your immediate supervisor, and what relationship is expected in terms of methods and frequency of communication?

3. How much direct authority do you have to make decisions? When do you need your supervisor's approval versus making a report of the decisions you made?

4. Will you need to develop personal goals in addition to program goals? How, when, where, and by whom will you be evaluated?

5. What performance evaluation system will you need to use with your staff? Are there different forms for different job categories?

6. What are the opportunities and regulations for hiring, promoting, and rewarding staff?

7. What are the regulations and guidelines for grievances or EEO issues?

8. What are the agency's basic policies (e.g., sexual harassment, emergencies), and where are written copies kept?

9. Are there any formal agency-orientation programs or requirements, and who should you see for what?

10. What are the policies and opportunities for short- and long-term training, continuing education, or administrative leave to attend professional meetings? What financial support is available?

11. Will time and support be given so you and your staff can meet with people in other agencies, divisions, and so on, to learn about their programs?

12. Is there an agency vehicle available for travel, or are you and your staff expected to use your own vehicles?

13. What systems are in place for ordering, purchasing, and paying for supplies, equipment, and other programmatic and administrative necessities? What forms and procedures are used, and who has signature power on accounts? What items need to be put out for bid?

14. How are telephone, mailing, and Fax charges made and tracked? What are the logistics of the phone system and for arranging conference calls?

15. What specific guidelines relate to professional and personal behavior and dress in your agency?

16. How are program income and expenditures tracked and reported? How many and which departments are involved with each part of the process?

17. What is the formal hierarchy of communication within the agency? Who can you talk to directly and when? Who are you supposed to contact via a higher level manager?

18. What is the mission and long-range plan of the entire agency?

19. How is the agency perceived by the public? Who are strong advocates and who are adversaries?

20. What management information systems are available for use by your program? What hardware and software are used, and can you expand the system if needed?

21. What federal and state workplace laws apply to your setting?

22. What divisions/offices (e.g., finance, personnel) are available within the agency for program support and employee support?

23. What are the policies governing use of leave (e.g., vacation, sick, without pay) and compensation for overtime?

**Figure 13.7**    *Questions for new managers of public health programs*

mulgation of rules and regulations. Individual agencies or programs then are expected to perform an enforcement role. Dental public health managers may be expected to draft or comment on legislative documents or provide testimony on issues such as tobacco use, fluoridation, Medicaid coverage, disclosure of HIV status, injury prevention, or budget reductions or program changes. As a result of laws passed, the legislature may request that agencies draft rules and regulations and hold public hearings for comments. Hygienists who have been active in legislative initiatives related to state practice acts or local community issues will be able to use these skills to understand their roles as agency personnel in the legislative process.

### Summary

This chapter is an overview of major issues that relate to management of dental public health programs. I have tried to incorporate discussion of issues that are not covered well in other texts or in most formal educational programs. Much is based on personal experiences and the premise "you learn the most from your own mistakes." The points that are never stressed enough are those we sometimes overlook when we are overwhelmed by the daily stresses and demands of trying to balance a professional career and a personal life. Specifically, if management of public health programs is so frustrating, why are so many of us still doing it?

It seems that many of the things we perceive as sustaining benefits are difficult to describe. The camaraderie and peer support among public health professionals is truly energizing and comforting. There is a high level of trust in one another's competence and commitment to improve health. There also is a high level of caring and respect for people no matter what their ethnic or socioeconomic identity. Competition among ourselves does not drive programs; cooperative efforts and sharing of information and resources are the factors that maintain services and activities. Cooperative research projects and conferences are the norm rather than the exception.

Many of us are lucky enough to be involved in diverse national or regional projects or committees that require extensive travel, exposing us to multicultural values and life-styles, thus broadening both our professional and personal perspectives. The friendships gained through this process often last a lifetime. One of the most rewarding aspects is being asked to share our experiences via presentations or texts such as this one.

### Review Questions

1. Find out what public health programs exist in your community and your state. Do they have dental components? If so, interview the dental director about management issues. How do the issues compare to those presented in this chapter?

2. Find a local public health program that does not have a dental component. Plan questions that would need to be answered during a needs assessment. Try to write a mission statement and at least five goals and objectives for a possible dental component.

3. Read an article in a dental journal that describes an oral epidemiologic study of a population group. Based on the data presented, outline a program plan for prevention services to various subgroups of the population.

4. Select a public health setting that interests you. Write a career development plan that will give you the skills and education to apply for a management position in that setting.

5. Create two different scenarios involving personnel problems in dental public health programs. Outline how you would handle these situations if you were the program administrator.

6. Pretend you have been given a budget of $100,000 to run a statewide health promotion program for senior citizens. In the middle of implementing the program, your boss tells you to cut your budget by 20% due to an overall state budget deficit. Describe how you would approach this problem.

7. You work for the federal government and are not allowed to lobby or directly contact politicians to advocate for the migrant agricultural workers whom you serve. How can you promote increased funding for dental programs for them?

8. You've been asked to form an advisory committee for a regional oral cancer health promotion initiative. What types of people or organizations should be represented on it?

## SUGGESTED READING

Entwistle, B. A., & Bruerd, B. (1986). *Contracting for services in alternative practice settings.* Chicago: ADHA.

Green, L. W., Dreuter, M. W., Deeds, S. G., & Partridge, K. B. (1980). *Health education planning.* Palo Alto: Mayfield Publishing.

Rakich, J. S., Longest, B. B., & Darr, K. (1985). *Managing health services organizations,* (2nd ed.). Philadelphia: W.B. Saunders.

Whitehead, K. D., ed. (1993). *Federal personnel guide.* Washington, D.C.: Key Communications Group.

Windsor, R. A., Baranowski, T., Clark, N., & Cutter, G. (1984). *Evaluation of health promotion and education programs.* Palo Alto: Mayfield Publishing.

Zarkowski, P. (1993). Community oral health planning and practice. In M. L. Darby (ed.), *Mosby's comprehensive review of dental hygiene.* St. Louis: C.V. Mosby.

## REFERENCES

Brown, W. S. (1985). *Thirteen fatal errors managers make and how you can avoid them.* New York: Berkeley Pub. Group.

Burt, B. A., & Eklund, S. A. (1992). *Dentistry, dental practice, and the community* (4th ed.). Philadelphia: W.B. Saunders.

Competency objectives for dental public health. (1990). *Journal of Public Health Dentistry*, 50, 338–344.

Hughes, J. T. (1978). Behavioral objectives for dental public health. *Journal of Public Health Dentistry*, 38, 100–107.

Johnston, A., et al. (1988). *Civil service 2000.* Washington, D.C.: U.S. Office of Personnel Management.

Nanus, B. (1992). *Visionary leadership.* San Francisco: Jossey-Bass.

Quick, T. L. (1990). *Unconventional wisdom, irreverent solutions for tough problems at work.* San Francisco: Jossey-Bass.

U.S. Department of Health and Human Services. (1991). *Healthy people 2000: National health promotion and disease prevention objectives.* DHHS Pub. No (PHS) 91-50213.

*Catherine C. Davis*

# CHAPTER 14

# Research

•━━━━━━━━━━━━━━━━━━━━━━━━━━━━━━━━━━━•

## Objectives

After reading this chapter and completing the review questions, the reader should be able to:

- List at least three possible responsibilities of a research manager.
- Describe the role of a clinical monitor in the pharmaceutical industry.
- Describe the role of a clinical research coordinator.
- Define institutional review board.
- Write a paragraph describing the role of an institutional review board member.
- List the eight essential elements that an informed consent document must contain.
- Design an informed consent document.
- State the importance of obtaining grant funding for research projects.
- Describe the role of a research manager in continuous quality improvement.
- Construct a career pathway to becoming a research manager, including identifying personal strengths, course work, and experience needed.

•━━━━━━━━━━━━━━━━━━━━━━━━━━━━━━━━━━━•

I remember the exact moment in dental hygiene school when I decided I wanted to be a researcher. It was the second semester of my junior year. I had just examined a patient who had some interesting pockets. He was a 27-year-old African American male who had 7–8 mm pockets circumferentially around all of his anterior teeth and molars. I thought, "Wow, I think this patient exhibits all of the signs of periodontosis." (Back in 1977, that's what we called localized juvenile periodontitis.)

I went to the periodontics department and asked my perio professor to confirm my diagnosis and treatment plan. He was excited about my findings also. I remember thinking, "I wonder what causes this disease? How can only these teeth be affected and why don't I see gingival inflammation and a lot of plaque?" My mind was racing a million miles a minute when my dental hygiene clinic instructor came over and asked, "What kind of brushing technique should we recommend to this patient?" I thought, "Brushing technique . . . brushing technique . . . Aren't you interested in finding out what is causing the problem? How can you recommend treatment modalities to intervene in the progression of the disease if you don't know what's causing it?" Of course, all of you are smiling at this point, because if you had clinic instructors like mine, who did not like to be put on the spot, you know that you couldn't say what you were thinking. I expressed my concern that a toothbrush bristle could not effectively reach the base of this patient's pockets to remove all of the plaque. Evidently, the correct answer was the Bass technique. (If you said that, you would have been right nine times out of ten.)

I took my demerit on my grading sheet and went back to thinking what could possibly cause this disease. If we are to be true professionals, shouldn't we know what causes disease in order to intervene with the proper treatment, rather than be technicians who "parrot back" the standard answer? From that moment on, I decided that I wanted to be in the forefront of determining what causes disease. Since that decision, I have faced many challenges and developed a discipline for studying and an enthusiasm for venturing into the unknown world.

## BACKGROUND

You already know that I decided during my junior year in college that I would not be satisfied in a traditional dental hygiene career. In high school, I thought that I would go to college, study dental hygiene, graduate, and go to work for a dentist. However, if there is any advice that I could give to an aspiring dental hygienist interested in being involved in conducting or managing research, it would be to have an open mind, educate yourself for the future, and network with colleagues.

By the beginning of my senior year, I had learned several things. I loved pathology, and I wanted to know why disease occurred. I needed to be in a challenging environment, but I had no idea how to find a challenging environment that would allow me to meet my future goals. I talked to some professors whom I admired, and one of them suggested a new graduate program for dental hygienists who wanted to pursue a master's degree (research based) in pathology. The program was located at Washington University in St. Louis. I had found the means to obtain my first goal!

The program was a challenge. I took all the oral pathology courses with the oral pathology residents and the statistics and research courses with the post-graduate dental students. My thesis research was completed at the Mallinckrodt Center, Division of Radiation Oncology. I conducted a research project that showed that high-energy electron radiotherapy followed by cobalt 60 for head and neck cancer could preserve contralateral salivary gland function compared to standard treatment. I had a wonderful thesis adviser who was a physician and would patiently explain methods of radiation therapy, critique my research design, and provide encouragement to keep going.

I learned many important things about research:

- Be motivated.
- Make a schedule
- Set realistic goals.
- Be able to work under pressure.
- Practice all analytical techniques before you use them on your samples.
- Complete all necessary paperwork.
- Get proper authorization to do research involving human subjects.
- Don't expect everything to come out perfectly.
- Have an open mind regarding results.
- Keep accurate documentation.
- Make copies of your lab notebook.

Toward the end of my two-year program, I had to start to think about finding a job to support myself. I thought, "No problem. I have a fabulous degree and experience. Someone must want my talent." I decided that I wanted to be in an academic environment so I could teach and design *and* conduct research. However, I ran into an age-old problem. I had nice academic credentials, but no job experience. I sent out more than 100 letters to various dental hygiene departments to inquire about jobs and got back at least 100 rejection letters, each containing the standard phrase "your educational background is excellent, but you have no experience." I could have stopped here, thrown up my hands and said, "I quit," but I didn't.

I found an advertisement in the newspaper for a part-time teaching position at a local community college and talked the director into hiring me. I also worked with my former thesis adviser to design a new research project based on the data from my thesis. I did this unpaid work on my days off, because I wanted the experience and wanted to work on honing my research skills.

In the meantime, Pauline Brine, from the University of Iowa, decided that she wanted me on her faculty and started recruiting me for the dental hygiene department. In December 1980, I accepted my first full-time job in academia at the University of Iowa, where I learned more about grant writing and conducting collaborative research.

Being a member of the University of Iowa faculty was fabulous professional experience for me. I was able to teach in a world-renowned academic environment with first-class researchers who were members of the Dows Institute for Dental Research. They all had different backgrounds; some were fluoride experts, caries experts, biochemists, epidemiologists, or experimental pathologists. I learned that it was important to attend journal clubs, be current in my area of research, estab-

lish a group of colleagues to consult with regarding research ideas, and fit
research into a hectic teaching schedule. Trying to set up a clinical trial can be a
challenge, since clinic schedules don't always match patient and clinician availability. But you must persevere and turn challenges into opportunities and make yourself do the work. I also learned the importance of bouncing ideas off experts in
the field. They had points of view and knowledge that I didn't. Again, cultivate
research colleagues. It is important for growth.

  After four years at Iowa, I also began to see that it was very important to have
credentials to do research. One of my colleagues told me that I needed a Ph.D.,
also known as the researcher's union card. This got me thinking. How could I go
on for a doctorate in science without taking a lot of prerequisites like physics,
organic chemistry, calculus? Someone said, "Why don't you get a degree in education?" I thought I would qualify but, all these people at the Dows Institute with
doctorates in science are the ones who are getting grants funded. Every researcher
must have funding to keep projects going. I was faced with a tough question. As in
undergraduate school, when I wondered how to get into research, I talked with a
colleague whose opinion I valued. He had two colleagues who were faculty members at Creighton University, in Omaha, and he thought that they could help me.
One was a physiologist and dean of the graduate school and the other was a
pathologist who taught at the dental school. He contacted them regarding my
interest in pursuing a doctorate in medical microbiology and getting a job teaching at the dental school. Talk about a dream being answered! I still consider that
chance meeting a miracle.

  After meeting with the Creighton faculty members, I knew that this was the next
path that I was going to take. The medical microbiology department waived the
requirement for physics and calculus, admitted me into the program, and gave me
a scholarship.

  I loved being in the medical microbiology department at Creighton. The faculty
was composed of medical doctors, who were infectious disease specialists and the
Ph.D.s who specialized in microbial toxins, antimicrobial agents, and molecular
biology. I took my first class with the medical students and was absolutely petrified,
but I learned so much that I couldn't believe it. I also took a course where we had
to present a research symposium. Guess what I presented for my first topic? The
pathogenesis of localized juvenile periodontitis associated with *Actinobacillus actino-
mycetemcomitans*. It was fun to explain to this group my full-circle encounter with
this disease, how in my lifetime the cause of the disease had been identified. The
defect in the host's immune system had been identified and a treatment besides
the Bass technique had been developed for these patients.

  The challenge that I faced was being in the laboratory. I had to learn how to
dilute, how to make buffers, how to work with the radioactive materials, how to
write grants, and how to keep with a project even when the results were disappointing. I did not do everything to perfection the first time. I made a lot of mistakes, but certainly learned what not to do.

  I also had the opportunity to present my research on the effects of alcohol on
the immune system to a variety of scientific groups, such as the American Federa-
tion of Clinical Research and the Interscience Conference on Antimicrobial

Agents and Chemotherapy. I got to network with researchers and talk with them on an informal basis. It was a wonderful opportunity. I thought that my next goal would be to do a postdoctoral fellowship in immunopharmacology, but as many married women learn, careers can take new turns when a spouse takes a new job.

When my husband moved to Fort Collins, Colorado, during the last year of my graduate education, I thought my professional life was going to end. However, the research attitude of not quitting when the results were disappointing that I had developed earlier helped to motivate me to find my next career opportunity. I knew that Dr. Irene Woodall was with Vipont Pharmaceutical, Inc., but I had never met her. When I contacted her to ask whether she knew of any positions, she was very kind and invited me to lunch to discuss possibilities. She didn't have anything to offer me at the time, but six months after that meeting, she called to ask whether I would be interested in writing the phase I and II reports for their new biopolymer that needed to be submitted to the Food and Drug Administration (FDA) for review. Vipont needed someone who was a dental clinician, microbiologist, and pathologist. My new career in the dental pharmaceutical industry was launched. After that job, I was offered a full-time position as the clinical and statistics monitor.

## MANAGING RESEARCH IN THE PHARMACEUTICAL INDUSTRY

My job at Vipont required that I design protocols to test the effectiveness of antimicrobial agents, irrigation, and other new oral healthcare devices. Once the protocol was designed, it had to be reviewed by the Protocol Review Committee regarding the ethics of the trial, since human subjects would be used (see next section on institutional review boards for more information). Dr. Woodall and I would develop a budget for the trial, select a research facility, and negotiate and finalize a contract to conduct the study. I would then go to the research site to make sure that the researchers were following the protocol. I loved doing this, especially when the trial involved microbial or immunological research.

I was required to review all published dental literature and keep the management and marketing departments at Vipont updated on current knowledge. I also worked hard to keep up on current findings in the disciplines of immunology and microbiology. I attended various research meetings to learn about new research techniques and how they would impact our products.

I thought I had died and gone to heaven because I'd found the perfect job for my skills and education. However, the economic situation in the early nineties forced the closure of our department and I was back to the want ads looking for a job for someone with my education and experience. Believe it or not, my current job appeared in the local paper. The local hospital was looking for someone to fill the newly created position of clinical research coordinator. They wanted someone with a Ph.D., who conducted research, managed an institutional review board (IRB), and could serve as a resource person to a variety of disciplines to foster research. I applied for the job and was hired three days later.

# MANAGING A RESEARCH PROGRAM IN A HOSPITAL SETTING

I was charged with the reorganization of the hospital's IRB and formulation of a multidisciplinary research support group. Since starting these two projects, I have also worked with the hospital's foundation to develop a research grant program and am currently learning about serving as a statistician for a new continuous quality improvement (CQI) program (CQI is also discussed in Chapter 5).

The first part of my job required that I participate in the reorganization of the hospital's IRB. The IRB had been operating under the authority of the hospital district board members and was changed to the authority of the chief executive officer. The IRB had been operating since the early eighties through the volunteer efforts of one of the hospital employees. The hospital's desire to encourage research necessitated that it hire a coordinator to serve as an entry point for all research.

Most of the research conducted at the hospital utilizes human subject data. Once an investigator designs a research protocol, it is necessary to obtain IRB approval of the research to protect the rights of the subjects. IRBs were established in early 1980s following public expression of concerns about the ethical conduct of medical researchers (Rothman, 1991). The purpose of this IRB is to protect the rights and welfare of human subjects participating in research. There are two points that an IRB must consider. The first one addresses the issue of the scientific validity of the study. Will the results gained from the study lead to the generation of knowledge, and do the benefits to be gained through the research outweigh the risks? Once the IRB decides that the benefits outweigh the risks to the subjects, the board must then decide what constitutes informed consent.

Informed consent is defined as a subject's voluntary agreement, based upon adequate knowledge and understanding of relevant information, to participate in research to undergo a diagnostic, therapeutic, or preventive procedure (Scannell & Ludbrook, 1992). The U.S. Department of Health and Human Services developed a guide stipulating the necessary components to be included in an informed consent document (USDHHS, 1983):

1. A statement of the nature and purpose of the research, the duration of the subject's participation, and identification of any experimental procedures

2. A description of the risks or discomforts

3. A description of expected benefits

4. A disclosure of alternative therapies or treatments

5. A description of the degree of confidentiality of subject records

6. An explanation of whether compensation exists or medical treatment is available if injury occurs

7. Contact persons for questions regarding subject rights, regarding the research, and regarding research-related injury

8. A statement that participation is voluntary and may be discontinued without penalty

Additional elements should be included where appropriate, including the following:

1. A warning that there may be unforeseen risks to the subject or to the embryo or fetus if the subject is or becomes pregnant
2. Anticipated circumstances under which the subject's participation in the trial may be terminated by the clinical investigator without the subject's consent
3. Any additional cost that may result from participation in the research
4. Possible consequences of the subject's decision to withdraw from the trial
5. A statement that new findings developed during the research will be provided to the subject
6. The approximate number of subjects involved in the study

I spent the first month of my job reviewing the Code of Federal Regulations that addresses the requirements for operating an IRB and providing informed consent. I reformulated the policies and procedures of the hospital's IRB and submitted the document to the chief executive officer and the chief of staff for approval. Once everything was approved, I sent out announcements of vacancies on the IRB, which now has four physicians, one nurse, one scientist, and two community members. I serve as an ex-officio member and consultant regarding federal guidelines. The chief information officer also serves as a nonvoting member of the group. They are a great group of people who serve voluntarily. We meet once a month to review protocols, informed consent documents, amendments, and adverse event notifications.

The IRB has reviewed several National Cancer Institute trials, the National Marrow Donor Program, and various new drug trials. We also have research that is designed by our own employees, such as a music-gait rehabilitation study for stroke victims and a study designed to test the effectiveness of reducing patient anxiety by the use of preoperative teaching.

One of the most important things that I have learned in this job is that it is very important to maintain accurate files and to create a paper trail that proves what communication goes on between the IRB and investigators. This occurs through recording minutes in a specific manner, acknowledging the receipt of all protocols, creating an agenda for the monthly meetings, and keeping computer records of all documents.

I review all projects before they are sent to the members of the IRB, ensuring that the protocols have the proper design and that the informed consent documents meet minimum criteria. Once the members review the documents, they convene a monthly meeting to discuss the project with the researcher. You can imagine that with the variety of backgrounds of the IRB members, we get many question. Very few applications fly through the IRB, and most researchers have to make modifications before the study can commence. I am also charged with receiving and reviewing the revised documents to make sure that they have been corrected.

I negotiate assurances with the Office for Protection from Research Risks regarding the review and approval of any studies that receive federal funding. I am very proud that our community-based hospital has made a commitment to research at a national and local level.

The second part of my job is to chair the Multidisciplinary Research Support Group. A variety of members serve on this group—nurses, physical therapists, occupational therapists, dietitians, medical technologists, and pharmacists. The group reviews all research that is designed at the hospital and endorses it before it proceeds to the IRB. We coordinate research between research groups. We have various tools available, such as a statistical package and a variety of computer programs, to aid in designing research, such as a program to help select the appropriate statistical test, design a trial, or assess the readability of an informed consent document.

We serve as contact experts in various subjects for people who have an idea about a project but don't know how to put it together. For example, two occupational therapists wanted to design a trial using a new neurological assessment technique to help them design appropriate therapies for stroke victims. It was important that they design and conduct a calibration protocol to ensure that they had intra- and interrater reliability for their research tool.

Research must be funded. Money is usually awarded through grants from various public and private sources. We are very lucky that the hospital has a foundation to address the needs of providing excellent patient care by purchasing equipment, supporting treatment programs, and awarding grants. I worked to start a small seed grant program for researchers to purchase nonexpendable supplies. These grants are awarded based on the merit of the project. The foundation has also supported several research projects designed by members of the hospital medical and nursing staff. Conducting research is a challenge and it is just wonderful that we have support to start small projects that are destined to become large-scale trials that can attract grant money on a national basis.

A third and timely issue that I am involved with is implementing a continuous quality improvement (CQI) program at the hospital. W. Edwards Deming, one of the patriarchs of total quality management, was responsible for the first sampling program in the country, used on the 1940 census and called statistical quality control. CQI, developed from Deming's ideas, is a data-driven management process that balances critical components of an organization, such as customer satisfaction, management expectations, employee fulfillment, and public approval. CQI is a focused management philosophy for providing the leadership, structure, training, and environment to continuously improve all organizational processes.

Our hospital management group has attended a variety of training sessions to help integrate this philosophy. We have devised flow charts, other diagrams, and cost benefit ratios and presented recommendations for improving operations.

I work with various committees to track the performance of a process through the use of statistical tools. CQI uses statistical probability rules and tools to distinguish common variation from special variation that can indicate problems. Statistics are used to identify, measure, and display output, defects, and distribution. These tools measure the effectiveness of a process.

## Summary

Little did I know that during my graduate education to become a scientist I would also learn skills that would make me valuable as a business manager in the future. As I stated earlier, it is very important to have a broad educational background and a variety of skills to be a marketable candidate for a job managing research.

## Review Questions

1. Describe the role of a clinical monitor in the pharmaceutical industry.

2. What is an institutional review board?

3. Write a paragraph describing the role of an IRB member.

4. What are the eight essential elements that an informed consent document must contain?

5. Design an informed consent document based on a protocol that will test the effectiveness of interdental floss versus interdental sticks.

6. Why is it important to obtain grant funding for research projects?

7. Why would a research manager be involved in continuous quality improvement?

### REFERENCES

Rothman, D. J. (1991). *Strangers at the bedside: A history of how law and bioethics transformed medical decision making.* New York: Basic Books.

Scannell, P. M., & Ludbrook, P. A. (1992). *IRB guidebook.* St. Louis: Washington University School of Medicine.

U.S. Department of Health and Human Services. (1983). *Protection of human subjects*, 45 CFR 46, 101-46.409.

# Index